A USER'S GUIDE TO BYPASS SURGERY

DATE DUE

DE __ 6'03			

DEMCO 38-296

A Note About the Author

Ted Klein is the owner of a pharmaceutical public relations firm based in New York and is the founding partner of MMD, Inc., a provider of contract sales personnel for the healthcare industry.

A USER'S GUIDE TO
BYPASS SURGERY

BY TED KLEIN

Ohio University Press / Athens

Ohio University Press, Athens, Ohio 45701
© 1996 by Ted Klein

Printed in the United States of America

Ohio University Press books are printed on acid-free paper ∞

00 99 98 97 96   5 4 3 2 1

Library of Congress Cataloging-in-Publication Data

Klein, Ted.
    A user's guide to bypass surgery / by Ted Klein.
        p.   cm.
    Includes bibliographical references and index.
    ISBN 0-8214-1143-8 (alk. paper)
    1. Coronary artery bypass—Popular works.   2. Klein, Ted—Health.
    I. Title
    RD598.35.C67K54   1996
    617.4'12—dc20   95-48908
                                                                    CIP

Designed by Laury A. Egan

Dedication

This book is dedicated to the memory of my late brother-in-law, James Stewart Kaufman, M.D. Throughout his life as a compassionate physician and for over fifty years of my life as his relative by marriage and as his sometime patient, Jim Kaufman was responsible for my care in countless ways. Most important for this book and the rest of my life was Jim's insistance that I continue to look for the reason for the "slight discomfort" that ended with a four-vessel bypass. It was Jim and my sister Joan who interrupted a trip to Russia and spent more than twenty-four hours traveling to be at my bedside just after my surgery. It was Jim who literally held the hands of my small family, offering information as only a family physician could. It was Jim's loving concern for me and my loved ones that brought us all through what turned out to be much more than an uneventful bypass operation. I wish he were still here to see how well I have done. More than that, I wish he were still here for us all to enjoy with him his amazing zest for life.

Contents

Foreword
by Robert N. Butler, M.D.

What a wonderful, valuable, and humane book is *A User's Guide to Bypass Surgery*. This work goes beyond the usual guide in its thoughtful depiction of the surgical act and the hospital-related experience of bypass surgery patients. Klein recognizes that the coronary bypass operation is not a cure and, therefore, he emphasizes undertaking lifestyle changes to avoid further cardiac problems. Each year, 400,000 people in the U.S. have a coronary bypass operation, popularly known as a "cabbage" (CABG), in which vessels are used to circumvent the patient's blocked coronary arteries. Over 30% of CABG patients are Medicare beneficiaries either over sixty-five or disabled.

Heart disease remains the number one cause of death, accounting for half of the two million deaths each year in the U.S. Half a million die from coronary artery disease. It would be useful, of course, if everyone got the message to live a healthy lifestyle long before a "cabbage" is necessary and switched to a low-fat, high complex carbohydrate, Pritikin-type diet accompanied by a serious physical fitness exercise program. Unfortunately, fewer than 10% of adult Americans fall into this category.

These years are marked by enormous turbulence in the healthcare system and the growth of managed care. This brings uncertainty as to whether patients will be able to obtain second and third opinions as proposed by Klein.

Furthermore, will patients have the right to choose their physicians? Klein recommends selecting a surgeon that has carried out at least 250 such operations each year.

Besides being an important guide for individual cardiac patients, this book can be read as a document with revolutionary potential in the area of medical patient advocacy. Indeed, I urge Ted Klein and others who have written useful books for consumers about a variety of diseases to become the founding parents and honorary chairs of an increasingly necessary American Patients Association, an organization that will defend Americans confronted with massive changes in our healthcare system.

Such a consumer organization has been overdue in any case. Too many people, old and young, are overwhelmed by the medical mystique which, along with institutional intimidation, makes it difficult for them and their families to advocate on their own behalf either in the doctor's office or in the hospital. In the fog of understandable anxiety, they may barely hear frightening information requiring life and death decisions. They are confronted with disturbing forms to grant permission for procedures and, perhaps, surgery. They may not even know or be told that there are lifestyle or medical approaches and not only surgical ones available to them.

The more sophisticated consumer may be armed by the *Merck Manual*, the *Physicians's Desk Reference*, and whatever books and magazine articles he or she may have read on a particular subject. But, in this era of the so-called information revolution and modern technology, there should be a wider range of rapidly available information tailored to specific situations that patients and their families can turn to.

It is time for people to take control of their own health and for doctors and others in the health provider system to recognize that they are, at best, professional "hired hands." The administrators and investors in various proprietary healthcare systems must appreciate that their customers have inalienable rights to comprehensive healthcare.

Increasingly it will be the primary care doctor who will decide upon diagnosis and referral. The primary care physician will have to become the specialist *par excellence,* a uniquely situated individual who possesses a comprehensive body of knowledge concerning a variety of conditions in order to both insure correct diagnosis and have the humility to know when to make the necessary referrals. Assessing the education and sophistication of such primary care physicians would be another job for the new American Patients Association.

A wonderful added touch to the *User's Guide to Bypass Surgery* by Ted Klein is a wise and sensitive commentary by his wife, Carole Klein, who experienced his medical/surgical experience with him. Since family members of cardiac patients are affected and become, in a sense, auxiliary patients, this insight into a spouse's experience wil be helpful to the husbands and wives of bypass patients.

If only more patients would write such valuable guides based on their personal experiences.

Robert N. Butler, M.D., is Director of the International Longevity Center, and Professor, The Henry L. Schwartz Department of Geriatrics and Adult Development, Mount Sinai Medical Center.

Foreword
by Thomas L. Petty, M.D.

Coronary artery bypass graft (CABG) surgery has been life-saving for many millions of people around the world. It can restore life's quality and improve the length of life. But CABG carries a mystique intertwined with fear, which can terrorize anyone, including doctors, who need this operation. Knowledge of the symptoms and risk of coronary artery disease itself ruins the bliss of the patient, other loved ones, and friends. It is bliss which is the foundation of a happy, productive, meaningful life, without which depression and despair result.

I have known Ted Klein since the introduction of nicotine-containing chewing gum as an aid to stopping smoking. His profound experience with CABG is a moving story, told firsthand by the patient. When he invited me to write this foreword, I was thrilled as I am also a member of the "Cabbage Club" (mine done urgently February 15, 1992).

Reading this powerful book, which has been extremely well researched for technical accuracy, along with the revelation of the patient's point of view, the de-personalization, uncertainty, and lack of consideration that, alas, permeates the modern medical system caused me to recall my own experiences; not all were pleasant.

Yet Ted and I have had the gift of return to health and the bliss that health offers. Everyone who reads Ted's book will be enriched, not only by knowledge, but they will feel a personal involvement in heart disease, the value of CABG surgery, a perspective on health maintenance as an alternative to disease, the recurrence of, and the emotion and experiences of a lovely and unique individual.

———

Thomas L. Petty, M.D., is professor of medicine, consultant, HealthONE Center for Health Sciences Education and Professor of Medicine, University of Colorado Health Sciences Center, Denver, Colorado.

Preface

If you are one of the 400,000 people who will undergo coronary artery bypass graft (CABG) surgery this year, I hope you will find this personal account helpful. I have always believed that knowledge and understanding give us more control over what happens to us. Doing research for this book has reinforced this belief, making me very conscious that if we have some control—any degree of control—it can make a major difference in the way we are treated in hospitals, even giving some of us an edge in coming through a potentially life-threatening invasive surgical procedure.

As a patient who has been told, "You need a coronary bypass right away!" you need to know a lot that I did not know when this happened to me. Given what I know at present, would I have done anything differently? No doubt about it! And I would have asked a lot more questions than I did. To begin with, if I had had an opportunity to read a book of this kind, I would have possessed certain knowledge, asked for additional information, and insisted on different care. My family would also have found me a lot easier to live with during my recovery from surgery.

When I was confronted with the recommendation that I have CABG surgery, I was told that I was a perfect candidate: a man at low risk for bypass surgery. (That's doctor language for "someone who has a good chance of coming through in good shape.") I had no history of coronary disease. At the age of sixty-two, I had never had a heart attack. Yet, despite my having chosen an expert cardiologist, a world-class surgeon working in a hospital with one of our country's best records for successful CABGs, I almost didn't make it out of the hospital because of two "unexpected incidents," one of which was life-threatening.

Now, five years later, despite my return to a full and active life, I am still very angry. I am still suffering from the psychological shock caused by the operations and the ensuing seven days in a cardiac intensive care unit (CICU). I keep waking up—often—because of God-awful nightmares. My right leg remains somewhat swollen as a result of the procedure which involved the removal of a fourteen-inch segment of saphenous vein that was used to make one of the longer bypasses.

I hope that some, if not most, of the psychic pain I suffered and still feel may be exorcised by the act of writing all this down. I also hope that reading this will enable my family, who suffered more than I in some ways, to learn how grateful I feel for their dedicated help, without which I would probably not have recovered. As it is, I am a healthy, active sixty-seven-year-old man endowed with a few, perhaps unnecessary, psychic scars. Those psychic scars are one of the major reasons I wrote this book. No one should be inflicted with their likes!

So what should a patient do? Read this book and learn all you can about your case and about the CABG procedure. After learning a few things the hard way, I also suggest that you request that your hospital assign you an ombudsman. Every bypass patient (and his or her family) needs an ombudsman to keep track of that patient's legal rights and also to deal with the family's emotions. I believe that if I had had such a person looking after me, I might well have avoided one or both of what physicians refer to as "untoward incidents." What I learned at the cost of considerable pain may help you get better care, with less suffering, if you are one of the thousands of Americans who undergo this year a coronary artery bypass graft operation.

While we are talking about information, it is important to keep in mind that the CABG is probably the number one money-maker for many U.S. hospitals. With that particular bottom line in mind, it is interesting to learn that experts disagree about how often a CABG is actually needed—knowledge that may encourage you to seek a second, or even a third, opinion. You should also know that the reason many CABGs are done is to "cure" anginal pain. Yet 40 percent of post-CABG patients experience a return of the pain as the grafted vessels develop new blockages. For example, Dr. William B. Kannel, one of the physicians responsible for the Framingham Heart Study (a multi-generational research program that studies the risk factors for thousands of men) is not at all sure that bypass surgery should be performed as often as it is. Recently he said, "It's fair to say it is not necessary to have an intense movement to surgery."

I wrote *A User's Guide to Bypass Surgery* to help people who may be facing this procedure learn something about what is happening and to let them gain some understanding and control over a crucial event in their lives—an operation which they may or may not need. The introduction tells you about my experience. I would like to hear from you if anything I said here was or was not helpful. I would also like to hear about your experience as a patient. I believe that there is a need for a patients' rights organization, an affinity group of CABG patients to act as advocates for everyone who has had a CABG. The Bill of Rights that is on page xxi will give an indication of what I learned that could help you.

Acknowledgments

I started writing this book in 1991, two years after I underwent four-vessel coronary bypass surgery.

There would never have been a book without the active encouragement, regular editing, and frequent literary conferences with my writing mentor, my muse, and marital in-house critic, Carole Klein. There were many others who kept me going. My cousin, Jordan Klein, called every day for weeks.

I had the idea for this book after reviewing others that had been written on the subject. To develop what I believed would be a unique approach to this medical story, I turned to friends and colleagues for advice. First, I thank Dr. Duane Schneider, then the publisher of Ohio Univeristy Press/Swallow Press. Had he not given me a contact, there would have been no book. Throughout the long writing process, Duane was very helpful in providing ample amounts of encouragement.

Also, Dr. Alan Lipschitz, my bicycle riding pal, deserves recognition for his council early on when he told me what I was writing was going to empower a whole generation of CABG patients. "You will give them that invaluable help that only knowledge brings. They will get better care and get better faster because of the facts that you have given them," he said.

Throughout my recovery, it was my children, William and Emily, who helped by standing by their mother who was constantly challenged by a patient-husband who continually doubted that he would ever recover his strength.

Countless friends came to my rescue. Joan Peyser called

to tell me that the surgeon that was going to operate on me did wonders for her. She kept in touch throughout my recovery. Louise Nett sent cards of encouragement from Denver throughout the early weeks and difficult months. Dr. Ronald Adelman came to the hospital to take me on my first post-CABG walk. His strong hand on my shoulder actually kept me vertical! Alan Fox called, and sent baskets laden with canned goodies and fresh fruits. We are still eating some of what he sent.

Charles Rongey came from Ohio to walk and talk with me. A client who became a close friend, his reassurance made me believe I could recover my business strengths as my body became stronger after the surgery. Soon following Charlie, from Sweden came Lennart Sorelius whose cheer brightened a bleak day in August that summer.

Stanley Siegelman, my friend for more than three decades, made a major contribution as my editor. If there is a tightness to this text, it is Stanley's hand that made it happen.

For the many whose gift baskets, cards and calls came over that recovering summer in 1989, both Carole and I say thanks. We continue to luxuriate in the glow of their love and attention.

A Bill of Rights for
Coronary Artery Bypass Graft Patients

Every patient with a coronary artery bypass graft (CABG) diagnosis should have the right:

1. To have the diagnosis confirmed by a second, or even a third, opinion.
2. To have a board-certified cardiologist explain in detail the nonsurgical alternatives to a CABG.
3. To have a partner, family member, or friend accompany him or her to hear the diagnosis that suggests a need for a CABG.
4. To have the hospital provide an ombudsman to represent the patient and the patient's family for the patient's entire stay in the hospital. (Very few hospitals offer this service. It is expensive and often can lead to problems for the hospital. Mount Sinai in New York has this service. There is even a graduate course in patient advocacy taught at Sarah Lawrence College in Bronxville, New York. I urge every bypass patient to ask if there is an ombudsman in the hospital where the CABG or any other major surgery is going to be performed.
5. To demand a medical team that has performed at least 250 CABGs the previous year.
6. To demand that the person who inserts the tube for the anesthesia should be a team member who has done 250 or more operations the previous year.
7. To demand a medical team that has a record of success with CABG procedures of 95 percent or better.

8. To be given a complete explanation of every step of the procedure, including how the patient may feel upon awakening in the coronary intensive care unit.
9. To have his or her family be told about the immediate post-CABG recovery period, when the patient could be angry and not entirely responsible for all he or she says.

A USER'S GUIDE TO BYPASS SURGERY

Introduction—A Memoir

My experience with bypass surgery began with a slight discomfort, not much more than that: a tightness in the chest one morning as I was swimming my customary half-mile at the New York University pool. I experienced just enough discomfort to make me get out of the water and start worrying. Three months later, almost to the day, I underwent a four-vessel bypass. This is the history of that coronary artery bypass graft (CABG) operation, called a "cabbage." I'll relate how I reached the decision to undergo surgery and some of the problems I had afterwards.

Three Months of Wondering or How I Decided to Have a CABG

In May 1989, I was sixty-two years old and weighed 190 pounds, about fifteen pounds overweight for a man five feet ten inches tall. I thought I was in excellent health. My family always thought of me as a jock because, for years, I would swim and bike almost every weekend, not to mention more often during vacations.

One Saturday, while swimming laps in the New York University pool, I felt that distinct discomfort—not pain really, just a tightness in my chest after swimming about a quarter of a mile. (I usually swam twice that distance.)

I got out of the pool and sat at the edge, thinking about that tightness. After a few minutes, I decided not to swim any more that day. I got dressed and, in the locker room, found myself feeling worried and very much alone. Why did I feel that mild discomfort? I knew the answer: it might well be the first sign of angina pectoris.

I knew that angina is often caused by a diminished supply of oxygen to the heart muscle. It is a common chronic heart disease. As a layman, I had fairly extensive knowledge of angina as a result of working in medical public relations for more than thirty years. Back in the early 1980s, my public relations firm helped to introduce Verapamil to the American medical community. This was one of the first of the calcium channel blockers used in treating angina and it became quickly known as a medical bypass. Thus, I knew what the symptoms of angina were and how it was diagnosed and treated. I also knew that no pill could cure the underlying condition which caused the pain of angina.

I dressed and biked the few blocks to my home. My head was filled with thoughts that made me extremely anxious. I knew I had to discover the source of my physical discomfort. I knew I must see a physician to find out whether I was suffering from cardiac disease. And if I was, I would have to look at my options. What treatment, if any, would be needed?

Before taking the plunge of making an appointment, however, I decided to give myself one more stress test. That was not such a smart idea. Why? Because it amounted to deliberately courting the risk of a heart attack. At that time, however, I did not know any better. Just seven days after my experience at the NYU pool, and without saying anything to anyone, I went on a strenuous eight-miles-in-sixty-minutes bike ride.

For almost an hour while I cycled, there was no negative repercussion. I felt excited and pleased. A week earlier, I had experienced discomfort while swimming, but, today, after subjecting myself to even greater stress, I was experiencing nothing of the sort. That tightness I had felt when swimming, I told myself, riding up the block to my home, was just a onetime anomaly. Forget your troubles! No need to worry. Then, just before I got home, the tightness came back. It occurred when I rode up a very slight incline. The feeling of tightness was accompanied by an attack of anxiety, underscored by a nagging, nervous feeling in my stomach. I was gripped by the fear of an impending serious, even fatal, illness. Once home, I did what anyone like me would do: I consulted my copy of *The Merck Manual*. Unerringly, I looked up *angina pectoris* in the index: "A clinical syndrome due to myocardial ischemia [a deficiency of blood supply to the heart muscle] characterized by episodes of precordial [over the heart] discomfort or pressure, typically precipitated by exertion and relieved by rest or sublingual nitroglycerin."

After reading this information three times, I felt very much alone and afraid once more. I knew that before me lay a slippery path with only two choices: denial or pursuit of the cause of the chest discomfort. I chose pursuit but did not tell my wife a word about my experiences swimming and biking. I did not want to worry her as much as I was worried.

Consulting a physician was the next logical step. I decided to visit Dr. Morgan (not his real name), my family internist, who had the records of my annual checkups for the past ten years. When I called for an appointment, his secretary asked if there was an emergency; I said no. (It may have been denial that kept me from admitting that, because I was so anxious, I was having trouble working and sleeping.) I was not scheduled for an appointment until about ten days later.

Nothing to Worry about

My family physician, who knew that I was in pharmaceutical public relations, greeted me with small talk and several medical insiders' anecdotes about his practice. Eventually, after what seemed to me a long period of badinage, he asked why I wanted to see him.

When I told him about the two episodes of discomfort due to exercise, he didn't seem to take much interest.

"But we should take an ECG (an electrocardiograph) anyway," he remarked as he asked me to undress for the examination. "After all, even a guy who is in as good shape as you are deserves to be checked out."

Minutes later, watching the needles scribble, he said, "Just as I thought. There is nothing, absolutely nothing, wrong with your heart. Get dressed and come into my office." There, he continued with his explanation for my chest's tightness and the discomfort from swimming and biking. In his opinion, the cause was either "an early touch of arthritis," or "probably muscular strain induced by stressing your body more than you should."

The second explanation, he said, seemed more likely. Either way, both diagnoses were music to my ears. He went on to tell me that I was about ten pounds overweight and reminded me that my hectic business travel schedule was "crazy." He reminded me that I had not had a vacation in a year. Besides, my daughter was going to get married in a few weeks and he thought this might be yet another reason for me to have tight chest muscles.

"But, let's put you on a beta blocker for a while to slow down your heart and help control that borderline hypertension we know you have," he concluded. "And please take it easy and call me after the wedding for an appointment." With that, he handed me a prescription for Lopressor.

In spite of his cheerful manner, my uneasiness persisted. "I'm happy you're not worried, but I am," I said. "I need to know, why the tightness? I want an exercise tolerance test."

"Why not?" he replied. He dialed the number of his favorite cardiologist—a colleague who, he said, was currently taking care of both of his parents. Within seconds, he asked the cardiologist to give me a stress test as soon as possible.

"As soon as possible" turned out to be just days before my daughter's wedding, so I postponed the visit until the week after. That was a week I spent in a state of high anxiety. I was afraid of what the heart test would show. Yet, in spite of the excitement of the wedding, there was no repetition of the chest tightness; on the other hand, I neither biked nor swam for the entire period before the scheduled visit to the cardiologist. You might say that I was denying any problem by not stress-testing myself with exercise.

My First Stress Test

On the day of my stress test, I ran for about seven minutes on the treadmill before feeling the same tightness in my chest that I had experienced twice before. When I reported this to the cardiologist who was giving me the test, he stopped the ECG machine, examined the printout and said, "Here it is." Pointing to the tracing, he explained, "The test shows that you do have a slight problem. You know what? I have about the same kind of ECG you do. And you know what else? I'll give you the same treatment I'm taking. All you have to do is take one Tenormin, a beta-blocker, twice a day to slow down your heart rate. You also need to lower your cholesterol, since our mutual friend Doctor Morgan told me that it's up to 250. I am giving you two Mevacors a day to take care of that." Then, ushering me to the door, he said, "Call me in about six months and let me know how you are doing."

He did not order a liver function test, listed as a warning in the material about Mevacor, which I read about later when I consulted my copy of the *Physicians' Desk Reference*. I don't like to take medications without reading about them.

Still, in a few days, the anxiety which had been very much a part of my life for weeks left me. I reasoned, "You were seen by a cardiologist, you were stress-tested, and he didn't worry. Why should you?" Nevertheless, I was still afraid to start swimming and biking. Two weeks later, I happened to talk on the telephone about my recent medical history with my brother-in-law, Jim, who is an internist. "You only went seven minutes?" he asked, sounding concerned. "How do you feel now?"

I admitted the pills were making me feel depressed and had slowed me down. That's not what Jim was asking about. Was I swimming and biking again without discomfort? I admitted that I was not exercising for fear that the discomfort would return. "You need to know more than you do about the reason for a physician to treat you with a beta-blocker," said Jim. He advised me to get another stress test, this time combined with a radioisotope scan. He told me that this test, with thallium-201 (a radioisotope), would show not only if there was a problem with the blood supply to the heart but also the extent and the location of any blockage which might have caused the angina.

"And then?" I asked.

"Then you will have a good idea about the next step."

"Which is?"

"You will need an angiogram to define the exact location or locations of the blockage. It could be that you have just one vessel blocked, and then maybe all you will need is a balloon to open it up," Jim reassured me.

In 1978, I had met Dr. Andreas Gruentzig, the Austrian cardiologist who created the technique of percutaneous transluminal coronary angioplasty (PTCA), in which a balloon is inserted and inflated to open up blocked coronary blood vessels. I knew this had become a routine procedure. Friends had told me of going to the hospital in the morning with angina, having the balloon inserted, and coming out that afternoon without any pain. I also knew that up to 30 to 50 percent of the people who had this procedure had a reoccurrence of the angina and therefore had pain after a PTCA.

A few days after my conversation with Jim, I spoke to Norman Isaacs, yet another physician who has known me for more than twenty years. I described my slight discomfort and the medication I was taking. "So, Bubby," Norman said, sounding concerned, "when will you have the thallium?"

I didn't have an answer that satisfied him. "I want to know just what is going on with the blood vessels that supply your heart," Norman insisted. "I will have my friend, Walter Steinberg (not his real name), who does thallium tests right in his office, do one for you." I said nothing. "So, we will talk," said Norman. "When you are ready, we will talk." He hung up. I knew I would be hearing from him again soon if I didn't schedule the thallium scan. Thus, I was faced with the next of many difficult decisions created by what seemed to me to be a no-win dilemma. I could listen to two physicians who had known me for years and schedule another stress test, this time with thallium-201, or I could stay with the advice of the first cardiologist who told me just to take the medication. Norman had said that if I followed that policy, I would never know if there was a blockage that caused the abnormal cardiogram.

I was still afraid to swim or go for a bike ride. I worried a lot about how long it would take me to learn to live with the side effects of drugs that made me feel so lethargic. I also worried about taking the next step, about finding out where and how extensive the blockage was. This information I knew might eventually lead me to have balloon angioplasty or even major surgery. I feared the latter the most.

Another week of worry ensued. I worried while trying to manage a busy schedule at work, including three day-long out-of-town trips. Each trip was marked by rushing to the airport and arriving late at every destination. Each arrival in another city was followed closely by stressful meetings. Still, I had no pain, no discomfort, just ceaseless worry about why I had the discomfort when exercising. That question wouldn't go away. I had to know.

Returning to New York from a one-day trip to Chicago, I had decided to call Dr. Steinberg to make an appointment for the thallium scan. Nevertheless, I postponed making the call.

The very next day, I got a call from the expert himself.

"Norman tells me you are a very close friend and not at all sure that you need the tests I give. Tell me about your recent problem."

Since Norman was not sure I would make an appointment, he had had Dr. Steinberg call me. Describing my medical history to the cardiologist took a few minutes, along with the recent episodes of discomfort from exercising and what I had been told by the first cardiologist; my brother-in-law, Jim; and our mutual friend, Norman.

"I agree with your two expert second and third opinions," said Dr. Steinberg. "Here is my appointment secretary." Seconds later, a cold voice told me to be in the doctor's office the next morning at 9:30. "Bring $850 and your exercise clothes and sneakers. And don't eat or drink anything until after the test. You will be here for an hour or so, then return three hours later for the final scan."

The worrying started again, along with a tightness in my stomach.

My Second Stress Test

This stress test was different. For one thing, it took a lot longer because of the thallium scan. I ran the same seven minutes before experiencing the same chest discomfort I had felt during the swim, the bike ride, and the first stress test. This time there was no immediate after-the-test consultation with the doctor. One member of his office staff (I counted three women in white behind the glass window) said, "In a few days, Doctor will send a report to your physician, and you will hear the results of the test from Doctor Isaacs."

This time, my wife, Carole, who was there with me, intervened. "No, we want to hear the results directly from Doctor Steinberg." There was a long pause. "I'll ask Doctor," the woman in white said as she left her protected area. She returned to tell us to come back the next day at three, when "Doctor will see you—and there will be an additional fee for his consultation."

Thinking about the results of a test that will tell you whether you need life-threatening surgery can heighten your sensitivity to details. Nevertheless, I am certain that Carole saw and heard more than I did late the next afternoon when we went to get the results of my thallium scan from "Doctor."

No longer dressed in his white coat, he sat behind decorator desk in a decorator office. His shirt and tie were both monogrammed with three initials. On his desk was a monogrammed sterling silver picture frame. I wondered if it would display a photo of his family in a monogrammed house. I was wrong; the frame held a simulated cover of *Time* with our doctor's picture on it. We waited for his diagnosis.

"There is no question about it. You have a major problem with several vessels serving your heart. As far as I can see, with the extent of the blockage, you have no heart muscle damage yet. However, I believe that you could have a stroke or a heart attack at any time. Do you keep nitroglycerin with you at all times?" The question sounded like a command rather than an inquiry.

"I don't have any," I answered.

"You should get some immediately," he said in a tone that frightened us both. "And," he continued, as he wrote a prescription for the drug I knew was used to treat anginal pain, "you have to get another test, an angiogram. I wouldn't wait too long to schedule it. Tomorrow would be good."

"Wait a minute," I heard Carole say. "Is there an emergency—a real cause to worry?"

"Yes, Ted could have a heart attack at any moment." He turned to me and said, "Don't schedule meetings uptown and then downtown the same morning or afternoon. Take it real easy. And be sure to carry the nitroglycerin with you at all times. Also, keep taking your beta-blocker."

Carole and I were both sufficiently frightened to ask him to make the appointment for the angiogram at once. I knew I was on that slippery slope, but I couldn't stop now. My life was threatened by the real possibility of a crippling or fatal heart attack. Dr. Steinberg reached for the telephone again.

"Who will do the test?" I asked.

"I don't know that," he answered. "It will be one of four people at Lenox Hill Hospital."

"Will you be there?" Carole asked.

"No."

I looked at her, she looked at me, and we both stood up at the same time. Unspoken but shared thoughts made us want to get out of that office. We didn't like that expert doctor. He was arrogant and frightening, not a person with whom we felt comfortable at this difficult time.

I could see he was surprised by our response. He stood up as we did and said it was up to me what I did with my life. We left. As we walked to the elevator, it was clear to us that I needed to find another cardiologist. Neither of us felt that this physician cared very much about me, and we both agreed that we wanted a physician who had good enough connections at a hospital to let us know who was going to insert a catheter into my heart.

The following week, I found out that the $850 I had handed over to the nurse was just for the test. The fifteen-minute follow-up consultation cost an additional $150.

The Search for a User-Friendly Cardiologist

What do you do when you need a cardiologist and can't ask either your family physician or the two cardiologists whose advice you have just rejected? I called my good friend, Bill Nelligan, who at that time was the executive director of the American College of Cardiology. (If you don't know Bill or someone like him who knows the nation's best cardiologists, I would suggest calling the nearest teaching hospital and asking to speak with the chairman or director of the Department of Cardiology. You have a good chance of getting the names of one or two cardiologists. For more information on how to find a cardiologist, see page 54.

I called Bill from our country home in Canaan, New York, on the Saturday after my unpleasant $150 consultation. He sounded interested in my story about the two cardiologists we had seen and rejected. Both were members of his association, he told me as he checked the college's directory.

"I know who can help you," he said. "And you know him, too—Simon Dack."

I knew about Dr. Dack because I have been a pro bono public relations consultant to Bill and the college since 1969. Simon Dack was the editor of the *Journal of the American College of Cardiology.*

Bill said he would call Dr. Dack and that I should wait until Monday to get in touch. Dr. Dack was retired, but Bill was sure he would find someone in New York to help us. He wished me well and gave me Dr. Dack's number. "Don't worry," Bill reassured me. "With Doctor Dack's help, you will be in the hands of the very best cardiologist in New York City."

Dr. Dack did not wait for my call. Minutes after I had talked to Bill, the portable telephone I had carried to our sunny backyard rang. "Hello," a very soft and gentle voice said. "Is Ted there? I am Doctor Dack." When I told him I was Ted, he asked me a few questions about what I had been told by the two cardiologists. I felt that I could hear him thinking. He said he would help me find someone, and instructed me to call his office for an appointment the day we returned to the city.

It was on a Tuesday, just three days after that Saturday-afternoon call from Dr. Dack, that Carole and I were sitting in a rather plush waiting room on the eighth floor of the faculty practice suites of Mount Sinai Hospital in New York. Promptly, within minutes of my scheduled appointment, a slight young man appeared carrying a medical record chart folder. He glanced down at the chart and up at me.

"Mr. Clean?" he asked.

"It's Klein," I said. My wife and I both stood up.

"No," said the young man, looking at Carole. "I just want Mr. Klein." He led me into an examining room.

"Take off everything but your shorts," he ordered, handing me a faded blue hospital gown that tied in the back, "and I will be back to get you in a few minutes."

"You don't understand," I began. "I'm not here for an examination. I'm seeing Doctor Dack to ask him to help me find a cardiologist."

Then I saw that there was no possibility of discussion. "I will give you a cardiogram, then take you for a chest X ray. Then you can see Doctor Dack," the young man announced before he left the room. I did what he asked.

A few minutes later, he returned to ask a few questions for what I could see was some sort of a patient record form. He weighed me, took my blood pressure, and gave me what was my fourth cardiogram in six weeks. Next, we walked to the end of a hall where an X-ray technician was waiting to take a picture of my chest.

Finally he took me back to the examining room and said my wife could now join us. I dressed and walked out to the reception area and brought a clearly anxious Carole back to the examining room. We waited in silence for not more than a minute or two before a very small man walked into our lives. It is difficult to explain. He had not said a word yet, but for reasons I still can't understand, I felt then and there that everything was going to be all right. Even Carole began to relax the moment he introduced himself. "I am Simon Dack."

Dr. Dack took my blood pressure, listened to my chest, and placed his stethoscope on both of my ankles. I had never been examined that way! Then he picked up the recordings from the latest cardiogram and told us to follow him.

His office was tiny with just enough room for a small desk, an office chair, and two gray, hard chairs facing the desk. There was a bookcase with just a few books, including the *Physicians' Desk Reference* and *The Merck Manual*. How impersonal, I thought and then remembered that this was a faculty office, undoubtedly shared by several members of the Cardiology Department.

"Tell me why you are here," he asked. He did not seem to be in a hurry, so rather calmly I recited my entire saga, starting with the slight discomfort in the NYU pool and the visits to my family physician and the two cardiologists. After that, I explained why I wanted him to help me find a physician with whom my wife and I could talk.

Dr. Dack looked at me for a long time. Then he looked at Carole. He began studying the records I had brought from my stress tests. Included were the letters from the first cardiologist to my family physician, the set of the tracings he had taken, the results of the thallium scan, and his report.

It must have taken Dr. Dack more than fifteen minutes to read through everything. We watched him in silence. He was completely oblivious of us and alone with his knowledge. He had spent fifty years or more looking at records just like mine. We will always remember how this small, elderly man, world-famous as the editor of a prestigious medical journal, studied my papers as if he had never seen anything like them before. From time to time, he would make a small sound and then write a note on a pad.

Finally I could not stand it any longer. "Doctor Dack?" I started with my most important question. "Whom do you recommend that I see as a cardiologist to take us through the next steps?" I knew what those were going to be and was beginning to become impatient. I was also a little miffed that I had to undergo yet another set of tests with the next doctor, who was likely to demand the same ones all over again. Most of all, as I watched Dr. Dack study my chest X-ray and the electrical and radioisotope records of my heart, I felt sick and old and very frightened.

He had not yet raised his eyes from my test results. "Doctor Dack," I said again, unable to stay quiet. "Whom will you get for my cardiologist?"

I wasn't prepared for his answer. "If you like, it will be me," he said, watching my face for a reaction.

I was surprised, and it must have showed. I had come expecting to be given a list of active physicians, not the help of a man who had retired. But there we were.

"Bill Nelligan says you need a cardiologist. You asked me for my help. You have it." With that, Dr. Dack looked at Carole, and gave her a sweet smile. In the same instant, we both agreed that he was to be my doctor. Thus began a relationship which no one in my family, most of all me, will ever forget. Suddenly things had changed. I was now his patient.

"Good," he said. "You have had very carefully done tests. I agree with the reports as I see them here." Dr. Dack was looking penetratingly into my eyes. I can't remember ever having been looked at as deeply as I was by this man.

"Most of all, I agree with Doctor Steinberg. The thallium scan is clear. You have major coronary vessels that are blocked."

I spoke, hot on his words: "And I need to have an angiogram." Then, because of our recent and very negative experience, Carole spoke for the first time. "Who, and when?"

The answer was immediate. "It will be John Ambrose, chief of the department. It will be done in this hospital, as soon as I can get him to do it." Dr. Dack reached for the telephone.

"This is Doctor Dack," he began. "I want my patient to be seen by Doctor Ambrose." A pause. "Good, he will be right over."

"Over where?" I asked.

"Over this way," Dr. Dack answered.

Dr. Ambrose was sitting in an office just as small as the one we had just left. He was dressed in hospital cottons and had a funny flowered hat perched on his head, as if he had just come from a child's birthday party.

The contrast between the two physicians couldn't have been more marked. I knew Dr. Dack was close to eighty. His colleague, the angiographer, was perhaps half his age, with his face defined by a black beard and an unmistakable twinkle in his gray eyes.

Because I knew this man was going to thread a thin tube into my heart, I found myself staring at his hands. They seemed as delicate a pair as I had ever seen. Dr. Ambrose noticed my concern and said, "I once was a fairly good classical guitar player. I even gave concerts."

"Did you ever hear the Romeros?" I asked.

"Great guitar players. Pepe may be the greatest living. But not such a nice man." I was won over. He could thread a catheter into my heart any time he wanted.

The entire conversation with Dr. Ambrose and Dr. Dack took about ten minutes. They weren't looking at me but at the reports I had brought to show Dr. Dack. Dr. Ambrose said, "I believe that you have no choice. You need to have an angiogram. I wouldn't wait too long if I were you."

A chill raced through me. "Call this number," he said, handing me a card. "We will do it next week."

The Angiogram

It was a very long week. I went to work in a fog and came home in a fog. A day or so before I was scheduled for the angiogram, I called Art Levin, a good friend who is a public health advocate. He directs the Center for Medical Consumers, a medical information service and library a few blocks from my office. "Because you seem to need to know more, you will find out more," he said after I explained my situation. "But I am not sure you will benefit from what you find out. Call me when you get the results of the angiogram."

The days went by. I still had no chest discomfort or pain, but I did not do anything that was in any way a stressful exercise.

The angiogram procedure is very simple, according to the receptionist who talked to me when I called to schedule my test. She told me, "All you need to do is check in at the hospital at about seven thirty in the morning. You will be able to go home about six hours later. Be sure to come with someone, since you will need some help to get home."

What she failed to tell me was that the examination has one possibly dangerous consequence and just four results. The danger in a very small number of cases, about one in five hundred—some patients start to bleed from the examination. The four decisions that are made as the result of an angiogram are (1) to use a balloon to open up the clogged vessels; (2) to do a bypass operation; (3) to implement a treatment regimen consisting of a rigid, low-fat diet, exercise, and (very often) drugs to effect a "medical bypass"; or (4) do nothing, since about 10 percent of angiograms are negative.

Physicians at Mount Sinai do about three thousand angiograms a year. Around 20 percent, or four hundred, of these show that a balloon can be used to open up the clogged artery or arteries. According to Dr. Ambrose, three or four of every ten patients have to have a second balloon procedure or elect to have a bypass operation. The balloon procedure is usually done several days or even weeks after angiography, unless there is some reason to insert the balloon catheter without any delay.

I entered the hospital early that morning, very apprehensively. Was I going to need a bypass operation? Could I get by with just medication? Would I be that rare patient who dies in the catheterization laboratory? These were the questions I kept asking myself. The issues came into even sharper focus when I was asked to sign a consent form which stated that Dr. Ambrose and the hospital were to be held harmless if I died from the procedure—in addition to giving the hospital permission to operate if the angiogram showed I needed a bypass immediately.

Minutes later, I was undressed, given a Valium injection, and taken to the catheter lab. At Mount Sinai, this is a large room equipped with several TV monitors and miles of wires. On a wall facing me, I saw a jumble of catheters hanging like white spaghetti wrapped in plastic.

The angiogram is done with the patient fully awake but sedated. I watched as Dr. Ambrose threaded a small catheter (tube) into a needle puncture in my right groin area. I could see a TV monitor above me. In a matter of minutes, I saw the catheter (it looked like a thin wire) move through a blood vessel into my heart. It was exciting to watch and I felt no pain, just a feeling of fullness in my chest. Then Dr. Ambrose called for the injection of a dye. He warned that it would make me feel very warm, as though my whole body had been dropped into a tub of tepid water.

A minute after the dye was injected, I saw what I had hoped not to see: several areas of visible blockage. I also knew the next chapter of the story: surgery, not balloon treatment.

Less than an hour after entering the catheterization laboratory, I was taken to a recovery room next door. A resident in cardiology began pressing on my groin over the puncture site that had been made to insert the catheter. Why must he use so much pressure? He answered it was because he had to be sure the hole was closed by a blood clot. Otherwise, I would start to bleed and this could cause a serious problem.

About four hours after I entered the hospital, I was ready to go home. I knew Dr. Ambrose would be studying the results of my test and was told he would report to Dr. Dack later that day or early the next morning.

I went to work the next day to keep myself from thinking about what I would hear in the afternoon when Carole and I had an appointment with Dr. Dack and Dr. Ambrose. Neither man looked very happy when we arrived. I knew what I was going to be told. Dr. Ambrose looked at Carole, then at me. "I have no doubt in my mind," he said. "You can't have a balloon—too many blockages. Most in places I can't get to. It's a bypass for you." I looked at them, then at Carole, and said that I wanted to think about it. We left the office.

For the next few days, I tried not to think about my need for surgery. I was in a self-induced fog. Carole tried to talk to me but could not get through. A cocoon of denial kept me from making the call to schedule the operation. I went on with my busy life and did not attempt any exercise. I did cancel an out-of-town trip, and I carried the nitroglycerin pills the self-important cardiologist had ordered for me.

Meeting Dr. Griepp

Less than a week after my angiogram, on a hot Thursday in June, I was sitting in a room at the midtown Marriott in New York City. I had just finished lunch with Bob and June Becker, two friends from Chicago. Bob is an allergist I had known for twenty years or more. The telephone rang. Bob picked it up. "Yes," he said, handing it to me. I was not surprised, since I always tell my office where I will be. This time, however, it was Carole. She didn't say hello. "You didn't tell me you had an appointment with Doctor Dack. He just called and is concerned that something happened to you. He is waiting to see us in his office."

"When?" I asked.

"Now," she said. "Call him and tell him we're both on the way." She hung up.

I called Dr. Dack, and he reminded me of an appointment which I truly must have blocked from my memory. I told him I thought I was supposed to call him to talk about the results of the angiogram and to discuss the next step.

"No," he said. "You were to be here today at two o'clock to meet me, and I have given your records to the bypass surgeon, Doctor Griepp, who has agreed to see you and Carole. Here. Now. Where are you?"

I explained and asked for forgiveness, promising to be in his office within twenty minutes. When I arrived, after a hurried trip across town, Dr. Dack was waiting for Carole and me in front of the elevators near his office.

He did not look like a happy man. "Where is Carole?" was his greeting. "We are late, so you have to come with me now. Carole will join us when she gets here." And we started walking very fast down long halls, in and out, and up and down two elevators.

Finally we reached a small but tastefully and carefully decorated office. I felt that here was the place of an important person. No name was on the door, but an elegant man sat behind the desk, studying a medical report I assumed was mine.

"Ted, meet Doctor Griepp," was my introduction. I knew who he was: a heart surgeon famous for successfully transplanting a heart, lungs, and a liver into the same patient. This accomplishment, several months earlier, had generated substantial media coverage.

Dr. Griepp was the first to speak. "You need bypass surgery. According to the angiogram by Doctor Ambrose, three, perhaps four major vessels are occluded and he will not be able to use a balloon to open them up."

I asked what my options were. Dr. Dack answered, "You don't have many. If you don't have medical or surgical treatment, we believe it is probable that you will have a sizable and, perhaps, imminent heart attack. We can't explain why it hasn't already occurred with the amount of blockage we see. We agree that you are incredibly lucky."

"The treatment you suggest?" I asked the surgeon.

But it was Dr. Dack who responded, in a soft and controlled voice. "As I said, you can choose between medical or surgical intervention. If you want to have the active life you seem to be accustomed to, it has to be surgical. And I want Doctor Griepp to be your surgeon."

With that, Dr. Griepp stood up. He told me he would answer any questions later, but since I had misunderstood the time of the appointment, he had to leave because "there is a room full of my residents waiting for me down the hall. You can stay here as long as you wish, Simon." Looking at me, he said, "If you decide to have the operation and want me to be the surgeon, it will have to be scheduled this coming Monday, since I will be taking a month's vacation the week after." He smiled, shook my hand, and got up to leave. I was very conscious that his hands would decide what would happen to the rest of my life. Dr. Dack glanced at me for some sign indicating that I understood the import of Dr. Griepp's words. Once again, it was not I but Dr. Dack who was the first to speak. "If Ted and his wife decide you will do the bypass, then what do we do?"

"Sally is across the hall. See her, and she will do the necessary paperwork," replied Dr. Griepp. Looking at his colleague and back at me, he said, "I'm sorry that I can't stay to meet your wife," and he left.

While he was sitting at his desk, I had failed to notice how tall and very thin he was. He had a distant look in his eyes, and I recalled his quiet way of talking. I also took in the watercolor of a large sailing ship on the wall facing his desk.

"He's going sailing next week?" I asked Dr. Dack.

"I guess so, he likes to sail," he replied. "But, you, what do you want to do? And where is Carole?" he asked, reaching for the desk telephone. "Has she come?" he almost shouted. "Yes, tell her how to get to Griepp's office." He hung up the phone, and looking at me, he said impatiently, "Let me go look for her." He walked out of the office, with me trailing after him.

We met Carole just as she got off an elevator. She had been lost in the maze of basement corridors that connect the hospital buildings.

The three of us walked back to the office where I had met Dr. Griepp and sat down, just looking at each other. I also spent time studying the picture of the sailboat. She was moving through rough waters, and I imagined I was aboard with Dr. Griepp at the helm. I continued to feel numb, thinking I was going to die regardless of my trust in Dr. Dack and Dr. Griepp. (That thought never left my mind until several weeks after I had come home from the hospital.)

Carole was clearly upset that she had not met Dr. Griepp. Dr. Dack was the first to speak. "If Ted is going to live an active life, then he has to have bypass surgery. I see no choice. And if Doctor Griepp is to do it, then it has to be this Monday. Do you both understand?"

Carole asked a few questions. I don't remember what Dr. Dack said. I just kept thinking about Monday. It was just three days away. Dr. Dack ended, "I don't think you should hesitate for a day. There is no good reason to wait. And with the extent of the blockage, you really don't have any options."

There it was. They would open up my chest. I was to have surgery in just a few days, or about ninety-six hours.

It seemed to me that Dr. Dack's voice had come from very far away. I heard the words "stroke," "heart attack," "operation," but they really did not get through. It was not that I wasn't listening; I just did not want to hear and have to believe what I was being told. So I stared at my shoes, then looked up at Carole's face. I do remember that Dr. Dack had a gold tie clasp placed rather high on his necktie.

None of us spoke much except that I heard myself agree to the operation. Dr. Griepp's scheduler was called into the office by Dr. Dack. She had obviously expected the call, because she knew my name and walked over to where I was sitting. "Give me a call later today, say about four or so, and I'll tell you what time you should check into the hospital on Sunday," she said. "I think it will be about five." That was it.

Carole and I walked out of the office and took the next train to our country house in Canaan, New York, to spend the days before my surgery with each other. I couldn't do much during the two-hour train trip except think about the trauma I would be facing. I had seen more than one film showing bypass surgery and could remember very clearly how the patient's chest is split open like a chicken ready to be grilled.

I managed to remember that I had to be sure Carole knew the location of all the papers that described my life and its obligations; the list was short, as I actually put on paper the information she would need if I didn't come home from the hospital. Then there were my two businesses, a small public relations firm which, nevertheless, had sizable assignments from several multinational pharmaceutical companies, and MMD, a national firm that provides flex-time sales personnel to the healthcare industry. What would happen to my staff? How would they be affected by my operation and recovery period?

I thought about Carole and our two children. What would they do without me? My only comfort was the knowledge that at least I would finally get something in return for all those insurance premiums. My small family would share over a million dollars. That thought did make me feel better; not less anxious, but decidedly better.

We got off the train in Hudson and I drove to our house in Canaan. I don't think Carole and I said very much to each other. I called my public relations office and told Diane Adams, who had been working by my side for twenty years, about my decision to have the operation in a few days. She was wonderfully understanding and supportive. "Don't worry," she reassured me. "We'll have everything taken care of here. Then I called Andrew Arkin and Barbara Saltzman, my two partners at MMD. They both reassured me that all would be well. ". . . not to worry. We will watch the store."

Di asked, "What should I tell our clients?"

I told her to tell most of them—all but one—that I was on vacation but could be reached in an emergency and that I would be back in the office in about a month. After that, I called the one client I had come to regard as a close friend and told him the news. He was just as calm and reassuring as Diane. "We'll have everything taken care of. Don't be concerned," he said. "You have spent almost ten years working for us, and we won't abandon you now."

The next three days were spent sitting in the sun, thinking about all the unimportant details of my daily life. I found myself taking an inventory of what I could see. The barn behind the house was redder then I had thought. The lawn was greener. My perceptions seemed sharper, but so was the intensity of my anxiety. I was on intimate terms with real, unconditional terror. I didn't talk to Carole about it. My defense when frightened is withdrawing into myself like a turtle hiding from the world inside his shell.

On the Saturday two days before my surgery, I got a call from Dick Morris, a physician friend of mine who had recently been through bypass surgery. Diane had told him about my scheduled operation.

"So you're joining my club," he laughed. "It won't be terrible. You won't remember any pain. There is one thing you should be prepared for, though." (This was a warning he might have stressed more, because acting on it would have made a great difference to me.) "The worst part of the whole procedure is that you won't be able to talk when you wake up in the recovery room because of the breathing tube in your throat."

If I had only remembered those words of warning it would have saved me frightening and agonizing hours when I awoke after surgery. You may well ask "Why couldn't you remember?" My answer is there may have been several reasons. Dick may not have made his warning strong enough. Also, the drugs that were used to sedate me may have erased whatever warning had been lodged in my memory.

That afternoon, however, I called Art Levin at The Center for Medical Consumers with some specific questions. What were the success and failure rates of the hospital and Dr. Griepp? "I'll call you right back," said Art, and in about ten minutes he was on the line with a good report: "Mount Sinai is as good a place as there is in New York. Only the Cleveland Clinic, two hospitals in Houston, and a few others have better outcome numbers. As for Griepp," he went on, "he is the number-two there, but the number-one is on vacation. You really can't do better than with Griepp as your surgeon and Dack watching out for you, Ted."

Some hours later, we took the train back to New York. To this day I don't remember a single detail of that train ride. I think I was numb with fear. From Grand Central Station, we went to our apartment on Tenth Street to pick up our son, his newly married sister and her husband. Then we went on to Mount Sinai, where at about five o'clock on Sunday, July 16th—just a month after my daughter's wedding—I began to fill out the lengthy form which is a key element of the hospital's admission procedure.

It seemed to me at the time—and it still does—that there should be a better way of dealing with a prospective bypass patient. The hour-long filling out and signing forms could be done in advance. Preadmission would have made matters much easier for me, allowing me just to give my name, show my insurance card, and check in. As it was, my family had to wait an hour (it seemed a lot longer) while I answered questions that a bored clerk read from a sheet of paper in his typewriter. Finally we came to the last question. "Do you want television?"

"Yes," I answered.

"That will be $4.50 a day, with a minimum of three days payable in advance."

I paid in advance. Just after he gave me the receipt, it hit me. "What happens if I don't come out of the operation?"

The clerk was not thrown by my question. "Initial here, and we will refund the total amount to your next of kin." He looked at one of the papers on his desk, paused, and recited, "That will be Carole Klein. You had best give her this receipt." At no time during that lengthy question-and-answer game was I shown the slightest bit of humor or empathy; nothing but a cold, by-the-numbers list of what is necessary to admit any faceless person.

I should have been prepared for this, but somehow I wasn't. Several months later, when I totaled up the bills of more than $95,000, I thought of the fun and pleasure that money would have given me if I had taken it and spent it on a first-class trip around the world. You know what I mean: only the best hotels; first class on planes, boats, and trains; excellent service. Instead, the only kindness and courtesy I got was from a dedicated group of physicians' assistants, one sweet intensive care nurse, and the great Dr. Dack.

My whole family went with me to X-ray, with me in a wheelchair pushed by an orderly. Fortunately it was a quiet night so that I was deposited in my room in less than an hour. One of the floor nurses handed me a hospital gown. Then came another shock.

"Please put all your clothes, your watch, your wedding ring, everything, into this plastic bag. You won't need anything for a few days, and we can't leave any of your personal possessions in the room tomorrow when you go up to surgery." The nurse spoke these words in a rapid, bored fashion. Obviously, they don't think I will need my razor, toothbrush, or watch because they aren't sure I will make it, I thought while handing Carole all my worldly goods. Taking off my wedding ring was most difficult; it had not been removed once since the day Carole put it on thirty-five years ago. I looked at my watch as I handed it over. Eight o'clock. I asked my family to go.

Just then a young woman, in a white coat that looked too large for her entered the room. She looked about twenty-five years old, younger than my daughter who was standing next to her.

"I'm Doctor Goodman, resident in anesthesiology. I have a few questions for you, and I will be happy to answer any you have," she said.

Our dialogue took about five minutes. She asked about allergies. I listed a few but none to anesthetics. I explained that I had no removable false teeth. She told me that I would be asleep during the operation for a minimum of three to a maximum of six hours or longer, adding the

promise "But you won't feel any pain, and you won't remember anything." Then she left.

I bid good-bye to a very worried-looking family. I could
sense plenty of free-floating anxiety. For them, and me,
the trauma was just beginning.

They left. I was alone. That's what I had wanted because
there was nothing I wished to talk about. I wanted it all to
be over. Three days would pass before I saw them again,
although they would be able to see me hooked up to a
respirator the following afternoon.

I turned on the TV, only to find yet another person
standing next to my bed, a woman who identified herself
as my nurse. "Wash yourself with this soap, all over twice.
It's antibacterial and smells funny, but it has to be used to
help prevent infection, you know," she mumbled. I know,
I thought, there is a good chance—perhaps 20 to 30 percent—that I would get a serious infection caused by a bac-
terium that I did not bring into the hospital. Yet another
cause for worry.

I took the bacterial soap shower, put on the gown that
opens in the back, climbed into bed and turned off the TV
set. I had a copy of a biography of Groucho Marx that my
son had brought for me, the one possession I had not put
in the plastic bag. I read for a few minutes and suddenly
felt very tired. I turned off the light.

The next thing I heard was, "Time to go. And let me give
you this injection." It was the same nurse who had brought
me the antibacterial soap.

"What time is it?" I asked.

"Seven."

I thought, It's 7:00 A.M., Monday, July 17. Am I going to
see Tuesday? I got the injection. I don't remember a thing
from a few minutes after that until two days later when I
woke up. I never saw the eighteenth; it was Wednesday,
July 19, before I had any consciousness of surviving the
operation.

I say I awoke on Wednesday, but I was not really awake.
I was in a twilight state. There was a terrible dryness in my
mouth, and I had an awful headache. My consciousness

was cloudy—so much so that I did not know where I was or why my mouth felt that way. Things got worse as my mind began to clear.

I couldn't talk; I couldn't move anything except my right leg. That was all I could do to attract the attention of a man who came over to the bed. I can still hear his words: "Don't beat your leg against the bed. I see you. I will decide what you need and what you get. You have nothing to say about what I will or will not do." With that, he strode away.

I could see that I was in a brightly lit room. Gradually, I realized where I was and then why I could not speak. I knew I had just had an operation, was in the intensive care room, and was alive. I did not know that it was Wednesday, that I had needed a second operation and was going to stay in that brightly lit room an entire week instead of the usual three or four days. I did not know what else was in store for me, but at least there was no pain. I slipped in and out of wakefulness like a light turning on and off. I was aware of other people looking at me, touching me, and then I saw my daughter's smiling face. "Hi, Daddy," were the sweet words I remember hearing from Emily. I was told it was Wednesday afternoon. It was the beginning of a nightmare of thirteen days of recovery, a process that usually takes half as long.

The reason for spending an extra eight days in the hospital was the second operation. It was necessary because a few hours after my chest was closed, it was discovered that blood was leaking—a result of a poorly closed blood vessel. This second operation traumatized my windpipe, causing me great pain, and almost resulted in the need for a tracheostomy, as I describe below.

My thirteen days' stay in the hospital were days neverending. Without visits from my wife, daughter, son, and son-in-law, it would have been impossible for me to keep any semblance of sanity.

When I woke up in the Cardiac Intensive Care Unit (CICU), I felt out of control and hopelessly unable to communicate: I couldn't talk because of the tube in my throat.

But, the brightest moment in that room, where they never dim the lights, came when I looked up to see a young nurse sitting at the foot of my bed watching me.

"Hi," she said, "I'm Marsha, your nurse, and I am going to sit here to see that everything goes well with you." She did just that for what seemed like hours. I still couldn't talk, but I did see she was caring for me. What she did I don't know because the CICU patient has literally no options. A machine breathes for him, bodily wastes are removed by tubes, other tubes feed him—and, yet, Marsha was there for me. Frequently, all she did was hold my hand. Her touch helped me with my fear, and for that simple act of concern, I will always be grateful to her.

Finally, the breathing tube was removed. I still don't know why the hospital hadn't given me a means of communication—a slate or a pencil and pad. I hope you keep this in mind and make appropriate arrangements beforehand if you ever go into surgery.

From the CICU, I was moved to the cardiac step-down unit with four patients to a room, every one of them monitored twenty-four hours a day for heartbeat, blood pressure, and other vital signs. Whenever some dramatic change occurred, a buzzer would sound in the nursing station to which all of us were connected. I remember the night one of the sensors connected to my chest came off. The buzzer sounded and in seconds, almost the instant I heard it, two nurses were standing next to my bed.

Being glued to the sensors, I had to lie on my back all the time. As a result, within a day of arriving in the step-down room, I began to feel the first hints of discomfort from what became a sore at the base of my spine (one of the infamous bedsores). After I left the hospital, it took two weeks for that sore to heal so I could sleep without pain every time I happened to roll onto it. (At the same time, I could sleep neither on my stomach because of the healing incision on my chest nor on my right side because of the fourteen-inch incision to harvest a vessel for one of my grafts.)

I did start to feel stronger in that step-down room, though. I felt a bit better every day. There was one incident, however, that persuaded me that I would ultimately get out of the hospital. One day about six in the morning, an orderly woke me from a sound sleep to weigh me. This made me so angry that I felt my heart rate increase dramatically. When the buzzer went off at the nursing station, I started to laugh because I knew the nurse on duty would come rushing to my room. Sure enough, she did, and found the orderly trying to roll me onto a scale. She must have heard me laughing, and a moment later, she, too, started to laugh.

"What's so funny, Mr. Klein?" she wanted to know, before asking the orderly why he was trying to push a patient who was hooked up to four different monitoring wires onto a scale. He couldn't answer. I continued to laugh. Being able to laugh made me feel that there was some hope—that I *was* going to get out of that room. It seemed clear that I couldn't be dying if I could laugh. Eventually I learned that my physician wanted to know my weight so he could judge my progress or lack thereof. Weight loss or weight gain is important as an indicator of recovery.

About three days later, on my seventh day in the hospital, I was moved to a private room. It had a TV set, telephone, and a private shower. My quality of life was improving.

Then came a second "unexpected incident." One afternoon, I began to have trouble breathing. My problem started with a dry cough, but as time went on I got the distinct feeling that my throat was closing. I was choking! I called the nurse, who called the physician's assistant on duty. She looked down my throat and explained that my cough was caused by a narrowing, a result of the trauma of the tube which had been used to anesthetize me for the second operation—the one required to stop the bleeding caused by the four bypasses.

A team of physicians led by Dr. Dack came into my room, summoned by word of this life-threatening incident.

Together with my family, they made for quite a crowd. Dr. Dack summoned the otolaryngologist on duty. Dr. Marvin Markowitz, who arrived a few minutes later, was very young and, I'm sure, had never taken the course entitled, "How to Reassure a Frightened Patient." If he had, he must surely have failed, because his first request was for everyone to leave the room.

As he began to examine me, I saw him set what looked like a plastic shopping bag filled with tubes on the table next to my bed. He saw me looking at the bag and anticipated my question.

"It's a tracheostomy kit."

My tight throat got tighter.

"Just in case," he continued.

I heard a very hoarse voice coming from a very sore throat ask why it was needed.

His answer was not the least bit reassuring. "You have a swelling in your breathing pipe. It often occurs with operations like yours. If it doesn't respond to treatment in the next few hours, we will have to open up your windpipe with the device in the bag. It will let you get air. If we don't, you will choke. It's as simple as that."

He looked down my throat for a few seconds, muttered something I did not hear, and left the room without another word. This bit of care cost my insurance company $850.

Two physician's assistants entered my room a few minutes later. Their concern was obvious; they were talking quietly and earnestly. One of them asked if I minded if she looked down my throat. I nodded my head in approval. She looked and said, "Prednisone would be worth a try." I found out later that Prednisone reduces soft tissue inflammation. For me, it obviated the need for a tracheostomy.

I will never forget that physician's assistant because—as I was told later—without that drug, I would have had a hole punched in my windpipe by that cold-faced otolaryngologist. As it was, in a few hours and after several doses of prednisone, I stopped coughing and started to breathe more easily. But that tracheostomy kit remained in my room until I left the hospital six days later. I was frightened every time I looked at it and took it home as a reminder of how close I came to having it used on me.

In spite of unanticipated incidents, I did survive hospitalization. Thirteen days after I was admitted, I left Mount Sinai, accompanied by my exhausted wife and went home to recuperate.

The Rest of the Story

I spent the last two weeks of that July in New York City. We paid one last visit to Dr. Dack, and off we went, for six weeks in August and September, to our lovely, quiet house in the country.

Approximately four weeks after the operation, I felt myself growing stronger. Carole would take me on an increasingly strenuous walk every day. Strenuous walk number one was all the way up and down the driveway. By the end of the sixth week, however, we spent an hour twice a day walking.

For me, the first few days were short. I got out of bed about nine in the morning and took a nap after lunch, followed by a walk, dinner, and bed. By the end of the second week, I was initiating and taking telephone calls. Visitors came; this made a great difference, not just to me, but to Carole.

My favorite client and good friend, Charlie Rongey, came to see me from Ohio. He took me for walks and enabled Carole to take a day off so she could return to the City for a brief respite from service as a nurse, exercise physiologist, and companion.

I was able to go back to work on a reduced schedule. Within a month, I could spend seven hours a day in the office. By late October, I was strong enough to leave New York for a two week visit to Rome and Venice.

Five years have passed since my bypass operation. I am living a new life. In a way, I feel this life belongs to someone else—the doctors, maybe. But, I think it really belongs to Carole, who willed me to continue living with her.

1

A Conversation with
a Cardiologist: Simon Dack—
How He Decides to Recommend
Bypass Surgery

The cardiologist who gave me the results of a thallium stress test made it abundantly clear that I was in "immediate need of an angiogram and probably bypass surgery" and that I should carry nitroglycerin tablets with me at all times. Then, just to make sure that I was completely unnerved, he suggested that I should not walk too fast.

His monologue and the way he delivered it, combined with his apparent enjoyment of the fact that the two people who stood before him were visibly frightened, was so cold and matter-of-fact, so devoid of human compassion, that Carole and I to decided he was not going to be my doctor.

Through a good deal of luck and the intervention of a close friend we eventually found ourselves in the consulting suite of Mount Sinai Medical School's Department of Cardiology in the office space reserved for the clinical teaching faculty. That is where we conferred with Dr. Simon Dack, then the editor of the *American Journal of Cardiology* and a world-famous cardiologist.

We knew there were few options: medical management

(with drugs and diet) or surgery. I also knew that my next medical encounter would be with an angiographer, since the thallium scan showed blockage in more than one of the vessels supplying blood to my heart. As I described in the introduction, Simon Dack became our cardiologist. He supported not only me but my wife and family through angiography, bypass surgery, an "unexpected" life-threatening surgical incident, an episode that almost led to tracheostomy, and finally, a process of recovery to the extent that today, I am in better health than I have been in many years.

Roughly three years after my surgery, I returned to Dr. Dack to ask him a few questions.:

TK: Dr. Dack, what makes you decide to recommend that a patient should have a bypass?

Dr. Dack: First, I want to know the symptoms. What is the patient experiencing? Why did he come to see me? Do the symptoms affect the quality of his life, his work, his daily activities?

TK: How do you do this?

Dr. Dack: By taking a history, then reviewing all the tests. It's the only way to do it. History's the most important thing. It leads to the decision for further workup.

TK: Then what?

Dr. Dack: There are noninvasive examinations that can be done that will give me information as to the severity of the underlying disease. If those tests suggest that there is multivessel disease that affects the patient's daily activities, then I would consider ordering primary angiography.

TK: You didn't mention exercise tests?

Dr. Dack: I did. Exercise or stress tests are noninvasive. I usually will start with just a stress test, then often ask that one combined with thallium be done.

TK: Do you feel that, without the thallium, they are useful? If you have a choice?

Dr. Dack: As an initial test, it is very useful.

TK: Even without thallium?

Dr. Dack: Yes. It's a good initial test because that's something that is relatively inexpensive and can be done in many cardiologists' offices. If that test is strongly positive, then I would certainly like to see a thallium test also.

TK: And then, when you've studied the results of the tests, what makes you recommend that the patient have either medical treatment or surgical treatment? What makes you decide between the two?

Dr. Dack: I'm not up to that yet. I'm up to the decision as to whether the patient requires primary angiography. I need the coronary angiogram to help me make a decision as to whether the prognosis, with just medical treatment, would be fairly good—or whether it's a high-risk situation and bypass surgery is indicated.

TK: What makes you decide?

Dr. Dack: If the patient's symptoms are well controlled with medical treatment, unless there is advanced coronary disease on the angiogram, I am willing to continue with medical treatment. Especially if it's one-vessel disease or two-vessel disease, prognosis is fairly good. Many cardiologists don't seem to realize that, if you have a patient with angina that's well controlled medically, his prognosis is fairly good. Mortality is not too high: one or two percent a year. Of course, if the patient is somebody who wants to be able to increase his activities, then you have to consider the surgery. If a patient tells me, "I'm not satisfied when you say I shouldn't do this and I shouldn't do that," then bypass surgery is indicated. If the patient is sedentary, doesn't seem to move about very fast, and I don't see any immediate threat to his life, I start with the medicines.

TK: So it's the patient who guides you.

Dr. Dack: Absolutely. The patient has to be involved. You can't order a patient to have surgery or not to have surgery. You can advise him. He makes the decision. Tell him what the prognosis is, the medical treatment, and tell him what the results would be with surgery.

TK: I remember you said to me, "To have the quality of life

that I think you should have, there is no choice. And once you decide that, you should have it done immediately—you shouldn't postpone it." Of the people that you've had this discussion with, how many of them chose not to have surgery?

Dr. Dack: About one-third.

TK: Have you followed up on these people? What happens to them?

Dr. Dack: Of those that I treat medically, some of them go along for several years; others have an acute cardiac event. You can't predict. I go on the basis of, out of a hundred patients like you, what would happen? But to you as an individual, I can't say, "Oh, within a year, this and this and this will happen." If I had a hundred like you, I can say within a year this is going to happen in five percent of the patients.

TK: As you know, there has been some criticism that, in this country, surgeons do too many bypass procedures. Do you agree?

Dr. Dack: It depends on the institution. I think most people here at Mount Sinai are very conservative. In spite of the fact that we operate on a good many very sick people in this hospital, our mortality rate is low. And very sick people have the highest surgical risk. I ask for bypass if the patient shows evidence of left ventricular dysfunction. That's when the heart is impaired because of the lack of blood supply. That patient almost always is a candidate for bypass surgery.

TK: What is the risk of not surviving bypass surgery?

Dr. Dack: I don't think the risk should be more than five percent at any hospital. If one takes sick people, it can be expected that they have a higher mortality rate than people who are not so sick.

TK: How often do you recommend a patient get another opinion?

Dr. Dack: There is no number. However, if a patient wants one or is told by the insurance company that he must have a second opinion, there is no question he should have it.

TK: How best should a patient go about doing that, in your opinion?

Dr. Dack: I think the best way is through his own family doctor or through the cardiologist who has made the diagnosis of coronary artery disease.

TK: You mean, ask the same physician, who tells you that you do or don't need treatment, to give you the name of another physician? Isn't there a natural conflict of interest? Wouldn't you expect colleagues to agree with each other?

Dr. Dack: Not necessarily. Perhaps it would be best to ask that a heart surgeon give the second opinion.

TK: All things being equal, to whom would you go—a surgeon or a cardiologist—for a second opinion?

Dr. Dack: Well, if I recommend surgery to a patient—I never do unless I review the angiography film with a surgeon.

TK: And you want to know why if he agrees with your recommendation?

Dr. Dack: And whether the surgeon believes that he can do the bypass effectively.

TK: *That* surgeon, not a surgeon.

Dr. Dack: Yes, the same surgeon that I would choose to operate on my patient. It all depends on how much you trust the physician. For example, in my hospital, if I have a problem making a decision, I call on a colleague here to review the patient's records with me, including all the tests that were done. Most important are the results of the angiography. I know I would get an unbiased opinion, even though we are very close.

TK: In your experience, when you are asked to give a second or—as in my case—a third opinion, how often does what you say confirm the first opinion?

Dr. Dack: About ninety percent of the time, and these are mostly consultations with patients not here in the hospital. This is often true if I know the cardiologist.

TK: That tells me a lot and is very reassuring. What happens when you do disagree?

Dr. Dack: I take the films and go to see the physician.

TK: You have told me that, in your experience, nine of every ten times, you agree with another physician's diagnosis. Yet you often recommend that a patient get a second or third opinion.

Dr. Dack: Absolutely.

TK: In your experience, how easy is it for someone who doesn't know anything about medicine and doesn't have a really competent family doctor to find a good cardiologist to help get that first, important opinion? My family physician told me to "take it easy, take a beta-blocker, and come back in six months." It was only after I insisted that I get a stress test and then a thallium that I came here and was operated on for four blocked vessels, a few weeks after I was told to "take it easy. . . ." What I am asking is how can, let's say, an unsophisticated patient, get to a Dr. Dack?

Dr. Dack: If a patient can't talk to his family physician, I suggest that he or she call the local medical society and ask for suggestions, but there is no best way.

TK: Once a decision has been made by the cardiologist and the patient to go for the surgery, what should the patient expect with respect to a continuing relationship with that first cardiologist, the one who recommended bypass surgery?

Dr. Dack: If a patient of mine is going to have surgery, I want to choose one of the surgeons here because, not only do I know all about them, I usually like to observe the patient during surgery.

TK: Why? Who needs you in the operating room?

Dr. Dack: It isn't that. I want to be there just in case I am needed.

TK: How many bypasses do you want a surgeon to have done before you make the recommendation?

Dr. Dack: The team does at least 250 a year before I make the recommendation.

TK: How can I tell if a cardiologist is the right cardiologist for me?

Dr. Dack: It's difficult. A lot depends on how you got to the physician. Who sent you? Was it a patient that referred you? Does your family physician know him? Have you checked his credentials at the hospital? There really is no best way. In the last analysis, if you don't have confidence in your doctor, you should look for one in whom you do. That is not asking too much.

2

Avoiding the Need for
Bypass Surgery

The landmark book *Prevention of Coronary Heart Disease* (edited by Judith K. Ockene, Ph.D., and Ira S. Ockene, M.D.) explains in great detail how physicians can guide patients at risk of death due to an early heart attack to a full and productive life. There is no way to provide you with a simple, short summary of this book, which is an important contribution to public health. I can only commend the Ockenes and their coauthors—and wish that my family physician had read some such book before I first presented myself years before I needed bypass surgery. "If only I had . . ." is a phrase many of us use too often. Nevertheless, *Prevention of Coronary Disease* should be required reading, not only for every physician but for everyone else whose family tree has had some branches cut short by heart disease. *Prevention of Coronary Disease*, if used according to its authors' intentions, should help reduce the number of wasteful and unnecessary heart disease–related deaths.

Coronary artery disease is a major public health problem. More than 3.7 million Americans were hospitalized for this in 1987. Approximately 37 percent of all deaths, or more than 500,000 people, die each year due to coronary artery disease.

Fortunately we can improve on these dismal statistics. New methods of diagnosis coupled with new kinds of treatment (including drugs and surgery) are already reducing those numbers, year by year.

In January 1991, the *New York Times* reported on the work of Dr. Joseph L. Melnick, a molecular biologist at Baylor College of Medicine. He hypothesized that a cytomegalovirus, a strain of herpes, may be responsible for causing the initial damage to an artery that will eventually be blocked with plaque. Thus, when scientists are able to develop a specific antiviral drug or even a vaccine, heart disease and heart attacks may be prevented.

My best advice to anyone who wants to avoid bypass surgery is to take great care in their choice of great-grandparents, grandparents, and parents; eliminate any link with every ancestor who ever smoked, tipped the scales at above-optimum weight, or suffered from diabetes, heart disease, or high blood pressure. Eliminating from your family tree any relatives who had strokes or heart attacks at an early age would also be helpful.

You say you can't do that? This may sound ridiculous, but it is also the best answer I can give you to the question of how to avoid coronary artery disease. Because your genes make it impossible to avoid this condition (at least, as of now, it is impossible to eliminate or change one's genome configuration), there is no way—brutally speaking —to avoid coronary artery disease. Even so, in being aware of potential risk factors (especially if you have a troublesome family tree), you can try to eliminate potential sources of trouble. In my own case, knowing that my father had hypertension and died of a stroke, I should have controlled my fat intake to keep my total cholesterol level at 200 mg/dl or lower (it was 260 before my surgery). I should have kept my weight below 160 pounds (it had been 185). I should have exercised daily, not just on some weekends. I never should have smoked.

Would these measures have spared me from bypass surgery? I'm not sure, but perhaps I could have beaten the odds a while longer and not have needed a bypass at age sixty-two. Knowing this, all I can say is, if you find yourself on a bypass track and experience angina, do all you can to find the best medical care and check out every bit of advice with a second or third opinion. If you elect to have the surgery, you will have to trust the skill of the surgeon and your body's great will to survive.

William Castelli, M.D., a member of the Framingham Heart Study team, is the first male in his family to live past age fifty. He knew that unless he took active control of his coronary heart disease, he would never make it to age fifty-one. According to Dr. Castelli, the only reason he has lived past his fiftieth birthday is because he watches what he eats and exercises regularly.

Taking a family history is one of the first things a conscientious family physician should do in the course of an initial patient visit. Michael A. Crouch, M.D., in his book *The Family in Medical Practice* writes that "the family is the missing piece of the medical puzzle. . . . The pure biomedical model of illness taught in medical school applies to only about 29 percent of what primary care physicians see in their offices." Most cardiologists will agree that a family history of heart disease, with one or more close relatives a heart attack victim, is reason enough to suggest an immediate lifestyle adjustment.

But you've heard this before. You know all this. So what is it that your physician needs to know before he or she recommends surgery? The answer is likely to be found in the results of a series of tests. That is true, even if the cardiologist, facing a patient who complains of chest pain after exercise (and admits her or his father, mother, and two brothers had heart attacks before age fifty), assumes this patient needs medical management and, perhaps, bypass surgery. That cardiologist will still go ahead and order tests. Below I describe most of them.

The Electrocardiogram

I assume you will have had at least one electrocardiogram

(ECG) already, but just in case you have not, allow me to explain how it is done and what its results (the most important part) can and can't mean.

A person who has had angina has at least a 50 percent chance of having a normal ECG. The test itself is painless, requiring just a few minutes. Although usually performed by a technician, the ECG is sometimes done by the physician, who attaches electrodes to your chest and legs. The electrodes are connected by wires to a device (the electrocardiograph) which records and displays electrical impulses from the heart muscle. Those electrical impulses are recorded on a narrow sheet of special paper. A trained individual can usually tell by looking at the printout whether the heart muscle is damaged in any way. A heart attack will cause damage to the muscle. The ECG indicates the extent of this damage.

When the coronary arteries are narrowed by 75 percent, too little oxygen-containing blood reaches the heart muscle. That results in a change in the muscle's electrical activity, which is readily apparent from the recording. That change is frequently, but not always, accompanied by anginal pain or reductions in blood pressure and pulse rate. If this occurs during the ECG, the test results are abnormal and the physician must decide on a course of action for coronary artery disease—either by medical treatment or surgery.

Sometimes an abnormal ECG is the result of medication (such as digitalis). An abnormal ECG can also result from deep and rapid breathing (hyperventilation) during the test. Thus, the results of one ECG test—normal or abnormal—should always be confirmed by a second or even a third test.

Since angina does not produce any permanent heart muscle injury, a normal ECG of a patient with angina will not be very helpful to the diagnosis. Mine is a case in point. And you, too, could well have an absolutely normal ECG if you went to your physician because of discomfort when exercising. The ECG test measures existing damage, but will not predict damage.

When I experienced the slight discomfort that led me to my family physician's office, I had a physical examination and was given an ECG by the physician's assistant. The doctor read the tapes and told me, "Your heart is sound; nothing to worry about. No need for any further tests. That discomfort you had that caused you to worry and made you come to see me? I'm sure that it came from stress—your crazy lifestyle of too much work and not enough relaxation. Maybe your discomfort started when you pulled a muscle while swimming. Take it easy, slow down, don't work so hard. And see me in six months." About eight weeks after hearing those reassuring words, I had four coronary artery bypass grafts.

Stress Tests

In my case, I remained uneasy even after the doctor delivered those comforting words. If the ECG is normal and your angina persists, your next diagnostic step is an exercise test (often called a stress test). So why not have a stress test just to see if there was any heart muscle damage that could have caused the discomfort? My family physician agreed and called a colleague to schedule one.

Stress tests are done:

· To evaluate the origin of chest pain
· To screen for ischemic heart disease (when parts of the muscle are destroyed by the lack of oxygen)
· To evaluate possible problems of heart rhythm abnormalities (dysrhythmias)
· To determine if there is a functional capacity disorder of the heart
· To help plan a rational exercise program (a fitness schedule)

· To determine the severity of heart disease
· To establish the effects of medicines given to control the symptoms of angina or hypertension
· To determine what damage occurred after a heart attack
· To provide an estimate of the risks of suffering a heart attack

An exercise test is valuable as a measure of fitness. This is why many exercise clubs and gymnasiums require one before a prospective member is allowed to use equipment that can increase heart rate markedly. Stress tests are also used to assess the results of cardiac rehabilitation. It is best to undergo a stress test in a physician's office, not a gym where a physician may not be present.

A stress test is usually not advisable when there is a possibility of unstable angina. This means that chest pain occurs while the patient is resting.

Many cardiologists do not recommend exercise tests for patients who complain of typical anginal chest pain because it does not provide a great deal of initial diagnostic information. This is a point on which experts disagree. For example, the American College of Sports Medicine (ACSM) recently revised its guidelines for preexercise screening of people with no symptoms of heart disease. These had stipulated that only men over forty and women over fifty should get a medical examination before embarking on an exercise program. But now, ACSM is recommending the test for all "high-risk" people (defined as people with hypertension or those who have had symptoms of anginal pain when exercising). In any case, *no one should take an exercise test without a thorough evaluation that includes a medical history. No stress test should be done if the subject has chest pain, high blood pressure, or irregular heart rhythm.*

Most stress tests are done on a treadmill, some cardiologists use a bicycle ergometer. An increasing number of tests on older patients, overweight patients, or those at some risk are injected with Adenoscan instead of exercise stress test. This medication causes the heartbeat to increase without exercise on a treadmill or bike.

Here is how an exercise test on a treadmill works: you run on the treadmill while the physician controls its speed and slope, increasing the difficulty of the exercise. Your blood pressure and heart rate are monitored continuously throughout the test, which takes no more than fifteen minutes. You will be asked repeatedly whether you have any pain or feel ill in any way. If you feel any pain or discomfort, you should report it immediately and the test will be stopped. The test will also be stopped if the physician notices any abnormal changes in your blood pressure or pulse rate.

If you do not experience pain or discomfort, the stress test will continue until the target pulse rate has been achieved. Shortly before my surgery, I ran for seven minutes to reach 142 beats per minute and did not report any pain, but my ECG had shown abnormal S-T segments (a measurement of heart activity that usually indicates the presence of coronary artery disease). Those S-T segments caused the cardiologist to stop the test and decide that I needed treatment. His recommendation was medical treatment with a beta-blocker and a calcium antagonist. Both of these drugs lower the heart rate, which the doctor said would eliminate the discomfort I reported when I was exercising. He also prescribed a medication to lower my cholesterol level. He did not interpret any of the tests he gave as indicating a need for bypass surgery. I know now that, if I had listened to that cardiologist, it was even money that I would have had a heart attack if I had continued my lifestyle of hardcore exercising mostly on weekends and vacations.

Stress Test with a Nuclear Imaging Agent

Also called a radionuclide test, this procedure is similar to the ordinary exercise test with one major difference: you run until achieving your peak heart rate, at which point the physician injects a radioisotope (in my case, thallium-201). The radioisotope is attracted mostly to healthy tissue. The first year after a heart attack, however, the scan will show the dead tissue and scars from other heart attacks. The exercise test with a radioisotope is accurate 90 percent of the time in diagnosing coronary artery disease. Stress tests with radioisotopes are significantly more expensive than regular exercise tests. The procedure is nonetheless often used and is the test of choice when physicians feel that the test will provide critical decision-making information. There are only slight risks associated with exercise testing. Even so, you should not take a stress test, with or without a radioisotope, unless you are under the care of a competent physician. You should not repeat the tests either just to see how well you may be doing. Unfortunately, many people take stress tests at health clubs, recreation centers, and gyms without competent medical supervision. People have suffered heart attacks when taking stress tests administered by some of the best physicians in the country. Acknowledging this risk, no competent physician would give a stress test without having emergency equipment and certain medications available if needed.

Multiple Gated Acquisition Test

The multiple gated acquisition (MUGA) test for coronary artery disease does not require exercise and does not involve catheterization. It measures the efficiency of the heart, also known as the ejection fraction. A normal ejection fraction of 70 to 75 percent indicates no heart damage, while a 25 percent ejection fraction is a clear call for medical intervention. The test is performed by injecting a radioisotope into an arm vein. Within a few minutes, a special camera will show images of the heart contracting. Those images are fed into a computer to generate a series of pictures of the beating heart which show the efficiency of the heart muscle.

Studying these pictures allows the physician to determine the existence and extent of heart muscle damage. In my case, this test was unnecessary, as the results of the thallium-201 scan were clear enough for the cardiologist to recommend catheterization the very next day. "You are a walking time bomb, and I don't think you can avoid bypass surgery," he told me. "The question in my mind is not if, it's when."

Other tests used in diagnosing coronary artery disease include

· Nuclear magnetic resonance (NMR) scans
· Echocardiograms
· Digital Angiograms
· Angiography
· Intravascular ultrasound

Angiography

Next to the exercise stress test, angiography is the most frequently employed test today. Getting an angiogram (*angio-* refers to blood vessels, both arteries and veins) is generally a walk-in, walk-out, one-day procedure. It will show if you have a blockage and where it is located.

During angiography, a catheter (an extremely thin tube) is inserted through a needle puncture in your arm or thigh and then threaded through a major artery into the arteries that feed blood to the heart muscle. When the catheter is in place (the test is performed on a sedated but conscious patient), the cardiologist injects a colorless contrast agent (often called a dye) that will show blockages of the heart arteries. The location and extent of any blockage is recorded on film, videotape, and digital imaging. Studying these images will enable a cardiologist or surgeon to decide on the next step: bypass surgery or angioplasty, an attempt to open the blockage or blockages with a special catheter equipped with a balloon tip. Lasers, miniature devices that act as Roto-Rooters and other devices are now being used. (A similar procedure is used in the diagnosis and treatment of blockages in legs, with angioplasty and bypass surgery.)

When I had this test, I was sufficiently conscious and capable of responding to questions from Dr. John Ambrose, a board-certified cardiologist who has made catheterization his specialty. I can recall watching the overhead TV monitor as the catheter was being threaded through a hole in my right thigh. It looked like a thin wire moving into the blood vessels that supplied blood to my heart. When the dye was injected, the blockage in four of my coronary arteries was only too obvious, and I knew that I would need to be treated surgically. Dr. Ambrose told us the next day that he was sorry to report that a balloon procedure was not possible for me because of the location of the blockage. My only choice was bypass surgery.

Between 10 and 30 percent of all patients who undergo coronary angiograms for chest pain are found to have normal-appearing arteries, according to a report at a recent meeting of the American College of Cardiology. Angiography is not without risk, but that risk is very small—about 0.2 percent, meaning that fewer than two of every one thousand patients who undergo coronary catheterization suffer a serious adverse reaction. Some will need an emergency bypass operation. After considering the alternatives (like almost half a million other people in 1989), I decided that the risk-to-benefit ratio was in my favor.

Half a million coronary catheterizations, together with 370,000 bypass operations and angioplasties, make these operations among the most common surgical procedures performed in this country. The number of coronary catheterizations has been increasing every year since 1929, when Dr. Werner Forssmann performed the first known angiography on himself.

Who should undergo angiography? I asked this question of John Ambrose, M.D., chief of the catheterization lab at Mount Sinai Hospital in New York. (His complete answer appears on page 76.) In short, he performs the procedure in almost every case when a physician requests it. He is careful to select only those patients whom he believes are good candidates for angiography. Working with a team that does three or more angiograms every day, he is confident about achieving successful outcomes.

The American College of Cardiology has published the monograph, "Guidelines for Coronary Angiography." The committee of experts responsible for this 1987 publication lists three main reasons for considering the procedure:

1. The presence during exercise of S-T depression greater than 1 mm but less than 2 mm
2. The presence of two or more major risk factors and a positive exercise test in patients with no known coronary heart disease (The risk factors are smoking, hypertension, hypercholesterolemia, positive family history, and diabetes.)
3. One or more prior heart attacks

The committee also recommended angiography:

1. After coronary bypass surgery, or transluminal angioplasty when there is evidence of damage to the heart muscle by stress testing
2. Before high-risk noncardiac surgery
3. In the evaluation of patients after cardiac transplantation

Dr. Siegfried Kra, in his excellent book, *Coronary Bypass Surgery* (New York: Norton, 1986), listed these reasons for cardiac catheterization when considering bypass surgery to treat the pain of angina:

1. If there is a strong suspicion of left main artery disease

2. If chest pain is severe and does not respond to medical treatment
3. If the patient elects surgery to treat his or her angina
4. If chest pain continues following a heart attack
5. If there is typical anginal pain, but the stress test and the thallium test are normal
6. If an abnormal stress test is accompanied by chest pain
7. If the stress test after a heart attack shows up abnormal

Dr. Kra says that cardiac catheterization should not be done or should be delayed:

1. If there is no chest pain, even if the ECG or the stress test is abnormal
2. If the angina is mild and responds to medication
3. If the patient elected not to have surgery
4. If the aim of the test is to prove the diagnosis of coronary artery disease (especially when the thallium stress test is abnormal)
5. If the goal is simply to study the arteries after a heart attack (if there are no further symptoms)
6. If there is an abnormal heart rhythm but no chest pain
7. If there is an abnormal ECG during a routine physical
8. If there is a heart murmur, such as that of mitral stenosis, that can be diagnosed with sound waves

Measurement of Blood Pressure Differences

In early June 1995 (June 13, 1995) science writer Jane Brody reported in the *New York Times* on a new test that may prove to be very important in predicting heart disease and stroke.

According to the article the test is easy to do, is inexpensive, and does not require any drug or surgery. Physicians compare the blood pressure readings in the ankle with reading in the arm.

Dr. Michael Criqui, a specialist in preventative cardiology at the University of California at San Diego was quoted as saying this test is in "a area of major importance." Since the tests "provide a measure of an individual's propensity for developing atherosclerosis, and that outweighs all other risk factors."

When I was examined by Dr. Dack in May of 1989, he was the first physician that ever used a stethoscope on my ankle. When I asked him why he was taking my blood pressure there, he said "sometimes I can hear a difference when I listen to your chest, compared to your ankle." He was ahead of his time.

3

Finding the Most Qualified and Accessible Cardiologist

In order for you and your family to survive bypass surgery with a minimum of physical and psychic trauma, the first thing you need to do is to find a physician who will act as your primary cardiologist and advocate. Bypass surgery and its alternatives involve life-or-death decisions, most of which you cannot make on your own. Even when you find this person, you may need additional cardiologists to give you a second (and even a third) opinion.

Why should you want a second opinion? There is still more art than science in medicine, and you want to make sure that you really should have the surgery. There is no way you can take a "test drive." The best you can do is to keep asking questions until you are satisfied with the answers. My cardiologist told me that, after being examined and tested, about one-third of the people who come to him for a second opinion decide *not* to have bypass surgery.

Before we go any further, if you don't have someone you can call in a medical emergency, you need to find that person now, before you start looking for specialists. To find a family physician, I would suggest asking friends, or even the neighborhood pharmacist (who is likely to know a great deal about local doctors), or call the local hospital and ask for the director of family practice residency. You can also call the American Academy of Family Physicians at (800) 274-2237 or the American College of Physicians at (215) 351-2400.

There is no established procedure for finding second-opinion doctors. You can ask your family physician for a referral, talk to friends, ask your neighborhood pharmacist, or call the largest hospital near your home and ask the director or chief of its Department of Cardiology for help in finding a cardiologist.

Most likely you are reading this book because your family physician has already referred you to a cardiologist. If so, you should consider checking that cardiologist's credentials.

Before your initial visit to the cardiologist, you should make a list of the questions you want answered. Then make another list if and when you see other physicians. It is worthwhile taking notes and recording answers so you can read what was said when you get home and are away from the excitement of the office. (You might even want to consider using a tape recorder, with the physician's consent.) Remember, you are the person who will be having the surgery. You have the right to receive answers to your questions, and the doctor has the ethical responsibility to provide you with answers you can understand.

Here are some initial questions to help you make an evaluation. If you decide not to ask them, perhaps your partner or family member can. If the answers don't seem frank and understandable or if the physician is not happy to take the time to answer in a kind and forthright way, you should look for a second (or even a third) opinion. It is *your* body we are talking about, not the physician's. See page 136 for the most-asked questions and the answers.

Questions for Your Family Physician

1. Why is he or she recommending this doctor?
2. Where was this doctor trained?

3. Can you have the name and phone number of one or two recently referred patients to talk to?
4. What does this doctor charge for the first office visit?
5. Where does he or she do the exercise testing?
6. What hospital does he or she work out of? This is important because the surgeon recommended by the cardiologist is likely to operate in the same hospital; if you choose another surgeon, your cardiologist is not likely to have visiting privileges at that surgeon's hospital and can't be your advocate after the operation.
7. Is this physician approved by your health insurer?

Just being in the same class at medical school or belonging to the same group practice does not mean much. These factors count, but they should not be decisive. If you are reluctant to ask your family physician these questions, you should probably look for another physician. You should not worry about embarrassing your doctor. By the way, don't ask where he or she would go for a cardiologist, since in my experience, physicians and their families often get the very worst care—and usually are the worst patients.

When I need to find a specialist, I consult my neighborhood pharmacist. Why? Over the years, I have found that pharmacists get to know a lot about physicians. They learn what kind of people they are, how much they know about medications, and—most important—how accessible they are to their patients and to the pharmacist. For example, the pharmacist knows if a doctor makes house calls and if he or she is the first (or the last) to try new medications.

If you have access to a library that keeps magazines, try to get a copy of the November 25, 1991, issue of *New York Magazine*, in which Janice Hopkins Tanne answers a good many questions about "How to Be a Savvy Medical Consumer." Even though the article was written mainly for New York–area residents, it contains a great deal of good information (much of which I have summarized).

Tanne recommends contacting the local medical society as soon as you have questions about a physician (noting that everybody who wants to be a savvy medical consumer needs answers to these questions). Medical societies are listed in the white pages, either under the city's or county's name. Better yet, call the American Board of Medical Specialties at (800) 776-2378. Inquire as to what specialty the physician is board certified in. If it is internal medicine or cardiology, you are on your way to uncovering the bare-bones facts about the person you are about to ask to help you decide if you need a bypass—and, if so, who it will be that will open your chest.

An even better way to get this information is to go to a library and ask for a reference book published by Who's Who. This multivolume work, *The Directory of Medical Specialists,* lists physicians by their specialties and the geographic location of their practices. It will tell you when and where they were born, which medical school they attended, the year they graduated, and the name of the hospitals where they interned and received residency. This directory will also tell you about a physician's hospital staff appointments and membership in professional associations, and whether he or she has a current medical school teaching appointment. Obviously, if your cardiologist and the surgeon she recommends are graduates of an inferior medical school, with an internship and residency training in a remote hospital with no medical school affiliation, your chances of having a first-rate medical adviser are not as good as they would be with a physician who went to a top medical school and was trained at a teaching center you recognize.

There are no guarantees, of course. The physician who attended a prestigious school could have graduated last in his or her class. Directory entries won't tell you anything about the physician's personality, either. Nevertheless, taking the time to check should help you in one way. It will begin to make you feel that you have some control over what will happen to you. I reiterate: gathering this information gives you understanding. This understanding usually gives a sense of control, and a sense of control may give you a better chance of dealing with some of the anxiety that is certain to come with surgery.

Once you have several cardiologists' names, I strongly suggest you go to a reference library and look them up in *The Directory of Medical Specialists*. If they are not listed, there is a good chance that they lack board certification. (You can avoid this if you ask your family physician to recommend only board-certified cardiologists.) In any case, if someone who has been recommended is not "boarded," that is bad news. Keep looking. When you do find that the recommended cardiologist is board-certified, take a close look at what he or she is doing, paying particular attention to academic appointments, meaning that Dr. So-and-so is considered accomplished enough to be entrusted with teaching future doctors. If you are not impressed, give some thought as to whether you want to place your heart in this doctor's hands.

The cardiologist you select is all-important because he or she becomes your quarterback, calling the plays that can mean life or death. These decisions include helping you choose the other experts whose advice and skill you will depend on, including a second (or in rare instances) a third cardiologist.

The most important question that will need to be decided is whether you need medical or surgical treatment. This book is written assuming that you are a candidate for bypass, but if you have not yet decided to have surgery, I strongly advise you to get more than one opinion. I got three before I found there really was no choice if I wanted to have a quality of life which for me involved daily exercise and occasional very stressful exercise (including scuba diving to a depth of 150 feet).

The information cardiologists need to decide if you need surgery or medical management starts with the medical history. Causes of illness or death in your immediate family are an important part of this history. If your grandfather, father, and brother or sister died at an early age from a heart attack or if you are a smoker, forty pounds over-weight, and suffering from severe chest pain, the examining doctor won't wonder too long about diagnosis. In such cases, an ECG plus the history can be highly accurate in telling the physician if the chest pain is angina.

Some years ago, a group of physicians in California tried out a computer program to diagnose heart attacks. Their study, which was published in the December 1991 issue of the *Annals of Internal Medicine*, concluded that a diagnosis based on physical symptoms, medical history, and ECG was accurate in 97 percent of the cases, whereas, emergency room physicians who based their diagnoses on what they saw (with no aid from the computer) were right 78 percent of the time. The final assessment in the diagnosis-by-computer was based on the analysis of blood levels of enzymes that are produced when the heart muscle is damaged. You would hate to be among the 19 percent missed!

We have already discussed the tests used in determining whether a bypass may be necessary. The results of these tests will help you and your advocate cardiologist decide if you need surgery.

Defining Accessibility/Sensitivity

When you call for your first appointment with the doctor that you might want to be your quarterback cardiologist, tell the person who answers the telephone how you got the physician's name. Explain that you want to see if he or she can help you decide whether you need bypass surgery as treatment for your angina.

If you have trouble getting an appointment or feel the person you are talking to doesn't really care about you or your request, look for another doctor. Why? Because if you have trouble making an appointment, chances are that you or your family won't be able to talk to this cardiologist when you need to. The busiest are often not the best. Being there and being available count a lot.

Should You Go to a Bypass Factory?

It stands to reason that the most skillful surgical teams would be those that perform the most bypasses. That, in fact, is what I found out. But should you leave home and go to one of these supermarkets of bypass surgery? A lot of people do. I would guess that most of them live in the smaller towns and cities whose local hospitals don't do enough bypasses to maintain proficiency in their surgical teams. So how many bypasses should a team do to stay in top form? My cardiologist said he wouldn't go to a surgeon for a bypass who doesn't do at least 250 or so a year.

4

Your First Appointment
with a Cardiologist and
The Next Steps

Take your partner or a close family member with you on this first visit. Why? First, you are likely to be a bit worried, perhaps somewhat agitated, and not likely to remember all the details that the doctor discusses with you. Also, unless both of you like and trust the physician, chances are that you may have real problems later when important decisions have to be made.

Stress Tests

Here are some questions you should get answered after you have had the first routine in-office ECG and the doctor says, "I think you need an exercise tolerance test, what many call a stress test" or, maybe, "I'm not sure what is causing that discomfort and pain when you walk up hills. It may just be a muscle problem or a touch of arthritis. Just to make sure, let's get the results of an exercise tolerance test." This is the time to inquire, "Do I need this test, or should I get a radionuclide or an echocardiography test, both of which, I understand, can be a lot more definitive?" Or, "What about using that new imaging agent Adenoscan? I understand with it, in conjunction with nuclear imaging,

I won't have to run on a treadmill." After that, find out who will do what test, where the test will be done, and how much it will cost.

Radionuclide scans (sometimes called thallium scans) and echocardiography tests cost about four times more than a simple exercise test. Both of these tests require a substantial amount of training and a sizable investment in equipment in comparison to what is needed for an exercise test. Most often they are done in a hospital. Is there a real difference between these tests? Depends on who you ask.

Many cardiologists have neither the equipment in their offices nor the experience to do radionuclide testing or to perform echocardiography. Many of them do have a treadmill or bicycle ergometer, however, enabling them to perform the stress test right then and there.

Some experts contend the radionuclide stress or stress echocardiography tests are overused. They say that one can make a judgment based on a clinical history and, if needed, the standard stress test. Patients are poorly positioned to get involved in this sort of technical dispute.

One of the points you may want to consider, though, is that cardiologists who do not have the equipment for a radionuclide or echocardiography stress test in their offices are not going to be paid for that test. Somebody else will. Many cardiologists insist that radionuclide or echocardiography tests are worth the extra cost to the patient. I believe every patient is entitled to an explanation of what each test can and can't show in his or her case—as well as what it costs.

I had already had an exercise test on a treadmill, and a radionuclide scan, when my brother-in-law, who was an internist, and another physician asked why I didn't have a more "definitive" test. After my first test, the results of which I received in the cardiologist's office, I got an on-the-spot diagnosis of "not much to worry about," and prescriptions for drugs to lower my cholesterol level and to slow my heart. I had a second test because of doubts about that diagnosis and treatment. Having the radionuclide test first would have saved me about four weeks of waiting before I was told that I needed bypass surgery. All of which leads me to conclude that, if your treatment is covered by insurance and cost is not a factor, it seems rational to start with the most definitive test.

You have the right to know, from the start, both the costs and the method of payment the physician will require. Some physicians will demand a check immediately after physical examination before giving the results to the referring physician. All will give or send you signed forms so you can be reimbursed.

Decisions about tests, however, should be made by the patient in consultation with the primary cardiologist. Remember that a negative or positive test result is not an absolute indication that your coronary arteries are or are not blocked. No one test is going to give absolute results, and no test will give you an iron-clad guarantee that you do or don't need bypass surgery. No test will assure you that medical treatment, instead of surgery, will guarantee you won't ever have angina again. Your clinical history and test results will give your cardiologist enough information to list your options, though.

When the tests indicate blockage of coronary arteries, or even if the clinical history of a patient is not definitive, a cardiologist may order an angiogram. Angiography is a surgical procedure, discussed in chapter 6, which shows precisely where and how much the patient's coronary arteries are blocked. Angiography is always done in a hospital and, even though the risk that something may go wrong is small, you would not want to be that one person in five hundred. Which means that, to be on the right side of the odds, it is best to select a cardiologist who does four or five angiograms every working day.

Computed Tomography

An experienced cardiologist I know tells me that ultrafast computed tomography (CT) is "worthless—a money maker." It is a new diagnostic technique, sometimes referred to as "mammography for men" by enthusiasts who believe it could soon become a routine procedure. Proponents of CT say that this test measures calcification in the coronary arteries. It takes around seven minutes but costs a great deal more because it requires a huge investment in equipment. Physicians who believe in CT believe it can show whether the pain of angina is due to calcium deposits in the heart as well as whether the patient is likely to have a heart attack. There are other experts, however, who doubt if the presence or absence of calcium is of any use in diagnosing coronary artery disease.

When You Get an Angiogram or Have to Consider Angioplasty

Depending on the results of various tests, you will be told whether you need to have an angiogram. If you don't need one, it's probably because your primary cardiologist believes you "can be managed" with medications. In that case, as long as you are comfortable with the recommendation, you can stop reading because you won't be having a bypass at this time. (Angiography was discussed on page 49.)

Percutaneous Transluminal Coronary Angioplasty

You may be told, after angiography, that you are a candidate for percutaneous transluminal coronary angioplasty (PTCA). About 500,000 of these procedures are performed every year, always in hospitals. Angioplasty involves inserting a balloon at the end of a catheter into a coronary artery. The balloon's inflation will open the blood vessel by squishing the blockage against the wall of the artery.

PTCA has a lot of things going for it. It is a short procedure involving a day or two in the hospital and an immediate success rate of about 90 to 95 percent. It is, however, not always successful and is not entirely devoid of risk. Between 1 and 2 percent of patients who have elective PTCA require urgent bypass surgery because the angiographer actually causes damage to the artery. After this sort of failure, bypass surgery is the only thing left to do.

Making the Decision to Have a Bypass

Very well, then. You've had your tests. You and your partner and your cardiologist get together. Here are the questions that must be answered now. Are you, or are you not, a candidate for bypass surgery? And, if not, why not?

Put another way: what are your options? What do you do if there is no clear indication for either medical management or surgery? What if things are iffy?

You won't need to be a physician to get the drift of a cardiologist's thoughts while considering answers to these important questions. You do, however, need to think clearly and be alert to nuances in the answers.

Suppose you ask, "What do you think I should do, now that you have the results of all these tests?" Quite likely your cardiologist will begin listing lots of options. You would do well to have a sheet of paper handy in order to record these so that you and your partner can talk about them later without wasting breath over what was said. Nothing resembling a satisfactory solution may be available, no matter what. Electing to postpone the bypass and opting for medical management may mean suffering a heart attack in the future. Choosing bypass surgery may mean the pain won't go away permanently because the coronary artery closes up again for reasons that are a subject of much dispute among experts. Most of those experts base their opinions on their own personal, clinical experience—in effect, from treating tens and hundreds of blockages, some of which may have many of the same characteristics as yours.

This dilemma is the reason I recommend getting a second or third opinion.

Questions to Ask Your Physician Now

1. What are the odds (if I decide to have a bypass or if I decide not to have a bypass)?
2. What are the medications you will prescribe, and how do they work? What are their side effects?
3. If I don't have a bypass now, what are the odds I will have to have one later? How much later?
4. If I have a bypass, how certain are you my angina will go away?
5. Will I be able to enjoy a full and active life, as I would define it, with the medications? Or with bypass surgery?
6. If I have the surgery, will there be a lot of postoperative pain?
7. What about money? How does the cost of anti-angina medication compare with the cost of surgery? Will I have to keep taking pills after surgery?
8. Whom do you recommend to perform the surgery?
9. Tell me about this surgeon. How many bypasses did he or she do last year?
10. What do you know about the success-versus-failure rates of this particular surgeon? (That may be "academic" to a physician but literally a life-or-death matter as far as you are concerned.)
11. Tell me about the hospital where that surgeon works. How successful has it been?
12. How many of your patients have you sent to this surgeon, and could I call one or two? (I know this is a difficult question to ask, but I did ask it and did talk to a patient who also happened to be a friend of mine and who was operated on very successfully by the same surgeon that Dr. Dack recommended for me. Her positive experience reassured me.)

13. What are my options? What do they really mean? (Don't ask, "What should I do?")
14. If I avoid or delay bypass surgery, what's the quality of my life going to be like with medical management?

5

Hold Everything! Get a Second Opinion—You May Not Need Bypass Surgery

If you live within commuting distance of New York City or are simply concerned, confused, and frightened by the bewildering variety of reasons for having (or not having) coronary artery bypass graft surgery, I would prescribe a visit to the Center for Medical Consumers in Greenwich Village. Appointments are not necessary, but you do actually have to visit this unique medical library since they usually don't accept phone queries. Its collection should contain the answers to many of your questions.

The Center is located at 237 Thompson Street, behind Stanford White's Judson Church, which faces Washington Square. This remarkable facility is the nonprofit brainchild of philanthropist Arthur Levin, who holds a master's degree in public health. It provides information free of charge to anyone who takes the time and trouble to drop by (Monday through Friday, 9:00 A.M. to 5:00 P.M., all year long). The telephone number is (212) 674-7105.

Once inside the brownstone, which used to be a private home, you will find yourself surrounded by stacks of books, a wall covered with medical journals, some tables with comfortable chairs, several file cabinets, and a copying machine. Everything is carefully indexed.

The Center publishes an excellent monthly newsletter called *HealthFacts*. Its October 1991 issue contains a well-researched review of current medical information about bypass surgery entitled, "Coronary Bypass Surgery: How To Avoid It." (Your local library may subscribe to *HealthFacts*; if they don't, they ought to.) Meanwhile, you can call the Center and ask for a copy. I believe there is a $2 charge.

Here is a brief summary of what *HealthFacts's* editor, Maryann Napoli, had to say about bypass operations. She concluded that up to 45 percent of these procedures are "either completely unnecessary or questionable." Her primary source is Thomas B. Graboys, M.D., who was then director of the Lown Cardiovascular Center in Boston, associate professor of medicine at Harvard Medical School, and also on the staff of Brigham and Women's Hospital. (The technically inclined can find his or her own report on the subject in the issue of the *Journal of the American Medical Association,* November 11, 1992.)

Dr. Graboys and his associates studied patients who had been referred for second opinions about the need for coronary angiography. The Lown Center researchers found that 80 percent (134 of 160) failed to meet the Center's criteria for angiography, 11 percent postponed the test, and the remaining 9 percent were dropped from the study for various reasons. "While there may be a limitation in terms of generalizing this experience to all patients with coronary disease," the authors summed up, "we reasonably conclude that an estimated 50 percent of coronary angiography currently being undertaken in the United States is unnecessary, or at least could be postponed."

Here is what Dr. Graboys told Ms. Napoli:

"A person who is generally well and has no symptoms goes for a screening exercise test and the results are positive (evidence of restricted blood flow). The person is urged to have heart catheterization (an angiogram). The person has the heart catheterization and is told, 'You don't know this, but you are sitting on a time bomb. You have two or three vessels narrowed. You must have an operation.' But, even if the person may very well have two or three vessels narrowed, he or she may do just as well on aspirin or a small amount of another angina medication."

In other words, beware of physicians who toss around "time-bomb" terms.

Dr. Graboys continued, "The key variable is how good the heart muscle is, not the narrowing of the coronary vessels. If the heart muscle function is normal, then all the large trials have demonstrated that there is no advantage of bypass surgery over drug therapy."

Ms. Napoli reminds us that heart muscle function is determined in two ways, by echocardiography or stress test. Echocardiography is an examination of the heart via ultrasound. As far as the more prosaic method is concerned, Dr. Graboys believes that, "If a person can go eight, nine, ten minutes on a treadmill test, then the likelihood of that person having a life-threatening disease is extremely remote."

A good number of cardiologists agree that a person with chest pain should seek a second opinion before agreeing to have surgery, but others disagree. However, many insurance companies now require a second opinion before they will pay for an angiogram and bypass surgery, the cost of which runs to tens of thousands of dollars.

My own cardiologist said a second opinion is needed when the patient thinks it is needed. When I asked Dr. Dack how often he agreed with the first opinion, he replied, "About nine times out of ten." I feel that a 10 percent difference is worth the effort and expense of getting a second opinion.

Whenever the exercise test shows some kind of problem exists, you will be told (more often than not) that you need angiography. An important question you should ask before agreeing to have an angiogram performed is, "What's the evidence? Can you show me that bypass surgery or angioplasty will prolong my life or prevent heart attacks?" You should also ask how medication or surgery is likely to affect the quality of your life, as you would define it.

Quality of life is one of those terms hardly anyone mentioned several decades ago. What is it, anyway? This is what Harry Wetzler, M.D., a senior scientist at InterStudy, a nonprofit health policy organization, had to say on this subject not long ago: "The most important (treatment) outcome measurement is the patient's quality of life. Quality of life has two dimensions: functional status and well-being. Functional status can be measured by reviewing how the patient responds to such questions as, 'Does your health limit you to walking one block?' and 'How often in the past month have you felt cheerful and lighthearted?'"

The only study I was able to find that described quality of life in patients after bypass surgery was in a 1992 article by a Belgium surgeon and some Israeli colleagues. Writing in the *Quality of Life Research,* the authors wrote, "Coronary bypass patients benefit broadly through a comprehensive rehabilitation program." I agree and must tell you that I was not given any formal program. It was my wife Carole who "rehabilitated" me. The twice-daily one-hour walks on the country roads in Canaan, New York, did it.

My own decision to have bypass surgery was made for one reason primarily: I was afraid of dying from a heart attack, or worse, being disabled by a stroke. Also I did want to stay as active as possible, defined (by myself) as being able to swim a half mile in twenty minutes, to walk four miles in an hour, and to bike several miles up and down the hills of Columbia County in New York, all without any pain or discomfort. I know now that there will be very little benefit ten years after my operation (in 1994, as I write this, I still have five to go), but I think the quality of my life has improved. Not entirely due to the surgery but due to the changes I have made because of the surgery. Could I have been managed with medicine, diet, and exercise? Perhaps. I will never know.

When what I thought of as "slight discomfort" reoccurred after seven minutes of running on a treadmill, I was told by my first cardiologist that I could very well just go on living on a low-fat diet and moderate exercise. As you may remember from the introduction, he told me I could expect to experience some anginal pain (as doctors would say) which would be minimized by two drugs he was prescribing, and perhaps this would have satisfied me, except for what I have to call a good bit of nagging from my physician brother-in-law and another physician. Most of you won't be so fortunate, but, as it was, both of them strongly suggested getting in touch with a second cardiologist and having a second stress test, with thallium-201.

The series of patients described in Dr. Graboys's article who did not have the recommended angiogram (and, thus, no bypass surgery) included very few patients who subsequently died of a heart attack. Over the next four years fewer than 1 percent per year died—even though they had been warned they were "sitting on a time bomb." What would have happened to them if they had had bypass surgery? No one knows. How many would not survive the surgery? Depends on where they had it and the damage caused by other risk factors.

Dr. Graboys and other critics of unnecessary catheterization attribute the increasing number of bypass operations to more than a single cause. No doubt about it: there are physicians who go for bypass surgery because they are scared of losing a malpractice suit: plaintiff (man, woman) has chest pain, ranging from mild to uncomfortable but not acute. ECG and blood tests have negative results, but the family physician doesn't want to take any chances. "Just to be sure," the patient is sent to a cardiologist. The cardiologist does a second ECG, followed by a stress test, again "just to be sure." Because the results are, well, ambiguous—in any case, not showing perfect cardiac functioning—our cardiologist orders catheterization. There are signs of blockage, so the patient is told, "You are sitting on a time bomb!" Bypass surgery follows. At the root of this scenario is the cautiousness of well-intentioned physicians who don't want to run the risk of being sued for malpractice; as they would, more than likely, if they didn't recommend surgery and the patient died from a heart attack due to a blocked main coronary artery.

No one knows—no one will ever know—how many unnecessary bypasses are performed each year. The overall number, however, is increasing. When asked by *Health-Facts* to discuss the reason, Dr. Graboys had this to say: "Every medium-sized hospital in the country is getting a cardiac catheterization lab because there is so much income from performing the procedure. So many hospitals are finding it difficult to survive without high reimbursement procedures."

Over the past decade, the number of coronary bypass operations has climbed dramatically. Their aggregate cost is estimated at $12 billion a year, or 2 percent of all money spent on health care in this country. My own four-vessel bypass at Mount Sinai Hospital in New York City cost over $95,000. This figure included angiography; visits to three cardiologists; fees of anesthesiologists, surgeons, and pulmonary consultants; private-duty nurses for three days of round-the-clock care; plus TV and other amenities.

Back in 1991, Medicare paid out $3 billion for 135,000 of the 350,000 or more bypass operations performed that year. This was second in total numbers only to cataract operations. The cost of bypass surgery, meanwhile, ranged from $21,092 at Ohio State University Hospital to $33,672 at Boston University Hospital, exclusive of the costs of diagnosis, from interviews to exercise tests to angiography.

Dollar figures can never tell the whole story, of course. Dr. Graboys feels that one must factor in "the fear of dying . . . fear of litigation." He decries "the public's obsession with heart disease when there should be an obsession with diet, exercise and stopping smoking." He contends that "we have trained too many cardiac surgeons and opened up too many open heart units. [Units that must] do a minimum number of cases, and if they don't they lose accreditation." In *HealthFacts*'s opinion, second-opinion doctors add to the rush to surgery because the second physician is often reluctant to disagree with a colleague (and, I add, social buddy). So what's the hapless patient to do?

A glimpse at what the doctors are being told may be of some assistance. Quite likely the best-read item in the March 1991 issue of the *Journal of the American College of Cardiology* was "Guidelines and Indications for Coronary Artery Bypass Graft Surgery." Everybody who may be facing this operation ought to study this report. It was put together by a task force of eminent cardiologists drawn from the American College of Cardiology and the American Heart Association. Your cardiologist will have a copy; so will most medical libraries. I summarize the task force's recommendations as follows:

For people who do not have any symptoms (like me, with a slight discomfort or what could be called "mild angina" when exercising) the task force says, "The coronary artery bypass operation is indicated only *uncommonly* [emphasis added] for asymptomatic persons with no or mild ischemia [heart muscle damage]. It is indicated when patients have important left main coronary artery stenosis [blockage] . . . and for those with severe proximal stenosis of a large left anterior descending coronary artery."

The taskforce recommends coronary artery bypass graft (CABG) surgery for patients with stable and unstable angina whose symptoms do not clear up after medical treatment. Persons who suffer a myocardial infarction (heart attack) may or may not need a bypass, according to the task force, depending on many factors. The surgery is indicated when coronary angioplasty results in complications and if the patient has already had a bypass. You would probably not have much choice when a CABG is indicated as a result of an angiography or because of renewed blockage after a bypass. The task force imposed no age limits but noted that anyone over the age of seventy-five is at a greater risk of complications during and after the operation.

What do *I* say? For two years after my CABG, I harbored a deep feeling that I had not needed the operation. While writing this book, however, I reexamined my hospital records (all three hundred pages of them) and talked to both Dr. Dack and Dr. Ambrose. As a result, I have become certain the "slight discomfort" that made me seek medical advice was caused by the blockage of four coronary arteries. Perhaps I could have avoided surgery by taking medication, but I am not sure I could have gone on riding my bike or continued to go scuba diving down to 150 feet along the Belize reefs. As I write this chapter, after my sixty-sixth birthday, I feel stronger than ever before. I exercise almost every day and have not had any chest pain or even "slight discomfort."

I believe it is true that bypass surgery treats only the symptoms. The surgeon who operated on me said, "I have only fixed the plumbing. You still have coronary artery disease, and unless you change your lifestyle, I will be seeing you again in seven to ten years." I have taken this advice to heart (to coin a phrase) and changed my lifestyle.

In my opinion, this is what it comes down to: if you are diagnosed as having angina and this opinion is confirmed by a second or even third physician and if your angiogram shows unmistakable blockage, you will need bypass surgery to maintain the ability to live an active life. I have no data to prove this, but the people I know who have avoided CABG surgery by taking medication do not have the same quality of life I am enjoying. At present, five years after bypass surgery, I don't regret it.

6

Conversation with
an Angiologist: John Ambrose

After my cardiologist, Dr. Simon Dack, had reviewed my previous test results, including two electrocardiograms, stress tests with and without a radioisotope, and chest X-rays, he told Carole and me that he wanted me to have an angiogram before making a decision about my treatment. When we agreed, he called Dr. John Ambrose to schedule an appointment.

Dr. Ambrose is director of the catheterization laboratory at Mount Sinai Hospital, where he supervises a team of cardiologists who collectively perform more than three thousand angiograms every year. He was selected as one of the best physicians in the country in a recent book by Woodrow White. My wife and I found him to be extremely kind and considerate.

What follows is the transcript of an interview with Dr. Ambrose that I hope will help you understand what an angiologist needs to know before suggesting a patient undergo bypass surgery.

T.K.: Dr. Ambrose, tell me what makes you decide to do an angiogram.

Dr. Ambrose: Almost always, it's in response to a request from a referring cardiologist.

T.K.: Can a patient call you directly?

Dr. Ambrose: Yes, but it doesn't happen very often. Most of my patients here at Mount Sinai, the hospital where I teach and work, are sent in on an ambulatory basis, as you were: in at seven o'clock and out the same day about five or six hours later.

T.K.: What are the advantages of coming in and going out on the same day?

Dr. Ambrose: There are several. One, it's a lot less expensive. And, today, when insurance pays for so many of the tests I do, expense is a factor. Also, most patients like the idea of losing only a day or two of work.

TK: What about angiograms that are done when a person is in the hospital under observation, perhaps because of suspicion that he or she may have had a heart attack?

Dr. Ambrose: Inpatient angiograms are done when a cardiologist wants to know the status of a patient's coronary arteries or, as you suggest, to determine the condition of a patient who has just suffered a heart attack or has, what we call, unstable angina. We do these to see if he or she has occluded arteries and could benefit from one or more CABGs. Or I may be asked to determine if the patient is a candidate for percutaneous transluminal coronary angioplasty, also called balloon angioplasty.

T.K.: Do you like to see the candidate for an angiogram before you do the procedure?

Dr. Ambrose: Yes. If at all possible, I prefer to interview the patient to get my own history. I usually also do my own physical examination, often order a chest X-ray, and sometimes an ECG.

T.K.: Why do you do all that? Hasn't the referring cardiologist done all those tests?

Dr. Ambrose: Yes, but since the patient is already scheduled, the reason I conduct my own examination is to determine if there is a sound medical reason *not* to do the test. In that case, I'll call the referring physician.

T.K.: What would persuade you not to do an angiogram?

Dr. Ambrose: The patient may be a little too old or in heart failure. Or perhaps I think the patient is either not taking the appropriate medication or is not taking enough of it.

T.K.: What are some of the other contraindications for angiography?

Dr. Ambrose: I am more reluctant to do an angiogram if the patient has a history of any kind of bleeding or kidney disease, because the dye we use in angiography to visualize blockage can make kidney function worse. But, in all honesty, while we might postpone an angiogram, if a cardiologist wants one, we usually do it. However, a well-trained angiographer has to be a good doctor. I don't just look at the arteries—I look at the whole patient. A competent angiographer not only is technically good but knows when to go a little farther, or when to stop, and when not to do an angiogram.

T.K.: How safe are angiograms?

Dr. Ambrose: Very safe or we wouldn't do them. In our hospital, for every one thousand angiograms we do, one patient may suffer an unexpected adverse effect. There is no question in my mind that the benefit of the procedure is worth the risk, but we do inform the patient of the risk and then ask that he or she sign a statement of informed consent. Without this permission, we do not do angiograms.

T.K: When do you recommend a repeat angiogram?

Dr. Ambrose: If, after bypass surgery or balloon angioplasty, the patient continues to have anginal pain, I recommend another angiogram to see if the bypass or the balloon was not successful or, in the case of angioplasty, the obstruction came back. I never forget that the reason for the bypass was that the patient was suffering from coronary artery disease. The surgery doesn't cure it. Unless the patient changes his or her lifestyle, eats a prudent diet, exercises, doesn't smoke and loses weight, it is likely the vessels that were used for the bypass will get blocked again. The return of the angina will indicate this. I usually will first ask that this patient have an exercise test with thallium. The results of this test usually will tell if an angiogram is needed. However, I don't believe that patients who have had a balloon or a bypass should wait for symptoms. So I recommend a thallium test be done in six months, and then every year or two, after a bypass or an angioplasty.

T.K.: If the test shows blockage, then what?

Dr. Ambrose: There are several options, including another bypass, new and experimental procedures like atherectomy, or more medicines. Above all, to avoid the need for another date with the surgeon, I strongly recommend that all persons who have coronary artery disease be very careful about their diet. In my mind, there is no question that you eat your way into coronary artery disease. The couch potato who eats a lot of food high in saturated fat and who smokes is on his or her way to a heart attack or stroke.

T.K.: Is there a good way to find a talented and experienced angiographer?

Dr. Ambrose: Yes. Find out if the angiographer does at least two hundred to three hundred procedures a year. One who does fewer is not one you should select. Obviously, there are a number of other things you should know about before you agree to have someone slip a tube into the arteries that carry blood away from your heart. You want an experienced angiographer. To me, that means he or she has had at least a year of specialized training after being trained as a cardiologist. For angioplasty, you want someone who has had a year of training in that procedure and is doing at least fifty a year. Also, you need not only an experienced angiographer but one who works in a place that has good equipment and also a good surgical team.

T.K.: How do you find this out?

Dr. Ambrose: The patient doesn't know, the patient assumes. You go into an established place, and the equipment is good. But that's important because you want to make sure the angiographer gets good pictures.

TK: Let's talk some more about angioplasty. On what basis do you recommend balloon angioplasty?

Dr. Ambrose: If the angiogram shows me blockage where

a balloon or some other technique like atherectomy will work to open it, and the patient and I agree that there is a good chance the angioplasty will be successful, I will do an angioplasty. It's really up to me, but unless there is an emergency, I always tell the patient and his or her family what I see and what I recommend. We talk and then the patient can decide.

T.K.: What are the odds that the artery will close up again (a situation known as restenosis) after a balloon procedure?

Dr. Ambrose: About three of every ten patients who have balloon angioplasty will be classified as long-term failures.

T.K.: Then what?

Dr. Ambrose: We have to talk with the cardiologist, the patient, and the family about the options.

T.K.: Such as?

Dr. Ambrose: Another balloon operation, a different intervention like atherectomy or a stent, medical management, or bypass surgery. There is no absolute way of knowing what you should do. Your best bet is to find a cardiologist whom you trust, and then take his or her advice. In my opinion, informed patients have the best chance.

T.K.: Thank you, Dr. Ambrose.

7

What It Will Cost

I will now give you some information about the cost of a routine coronary artery bypass graft operation. Note the word *routine*. Obviously, there are no routine operations when it comes to your body. The issue will look different to a surgeon who does two or three operations a day at a hospital where five hundred or more CABGs are done every year. Most of these operations will come to appear routine. The surgeons at Mount Sinai told me that my operation was expected to be routine ("You will be out of the hospital in a week, back at work in six weeks or even less"), only an "unforeseen incident" changed things so that I spent thirteen days in the hospital and did not get back to work—part-time—until eight weeks later.

My nonroutine operation cost my insurance carriers a total of $95,000. This included all my pre-surgical work-ups—appointments with my family physician, three cardiologists, a variety of tests, an anesthesiologist, a surgeon who performed a four-coronary-artery-bypass operation, thirteen days in the hospital, two consultations with an otolaryngologist, twice-a-day visits in the hospital by my cardiologist, and two home visits by a practical nurse (to change a dressing).

My neighbor, Charles, had a four-vessel bypass a few days before mine at a hospital in Atlanta. His total bill was about $15,000. Five years later we both are in about the same shape. We compare our health regularly, and we can't see any difference in the outcome for our operations. It seems to me that Charles's insurance company got a much better deal than did mine!

What will your operation cost you or your insurance company? Can you shop for the best price? I can't give a definitive answer to the first question, but the answer to the second question is a definite, Yes! You can shop around, not only for the best surgeon (which I would define as "very well qualified") but also for a best buy. This will require a little homework, including—yes—comparison shopping.

If you are planning to have a CABG, be sure to contact every one of your insurance carriers to get an authorization number or whatever the hospital asks you to get before the surgery is scheduled. You don't need the hassle of payment confusion when you are ready to check out of the hospital. Keep all your insurance information handy.

My research for this chapter included contact with the Health Care Finance Administration (HCFA), which administers Medicare. In 1991, HCFA paid $3 billion for 135,000 bypass operations. The costs was about $21,000 (Ohio State University Hospital) to about $33,500 (Boston's University Hospital.)

8

Percutaneous Transluminal Coronary Angioplasty and Other Alternatives to Bypass Surgery

Over 420,000 percutaneous transluminal coronary angioplasties (PTCAs) are performed each year, making PTCAs one of the most common surgical procedures performed in this country. Angioplasty is used as an alternative to bypass surgery and is a less risky treatment for blocked coronary arteries. The procedure can also be used to open blocked blood vessels in other parts of the body.

Coronary angioplasty was first performed in 1977 and later perfected by Dr. Andreas Gruentzig in Switzerland at Zurich Medical College. It employs the same technique as coronary catheterization except that a tiny balloon is placed at the end of the catheter. The balloon can be inflated when the angiographer, watching via fluoroscopy, sees that an artery is blocked. As the balloon expands, the plaque that has been blocking the artery is pushed into the wall of the artery, opening up the vessel and allowing blood to flow.

The immediate success rate of angioplasty has now reached 90 percent in many hospitals and 95 percent in centers specializing in the procedure. As you might expect, the results of the operation depend on several factors, mainly the skill of the surgical team, the health of the patient, and the extent and characteristics of the athero-sclerotic plaque that is impeding blood flow. The likelihood of success is greatest with male patients under the age of 65 who have normal ventricular function and one or two accessible blocked vessels. If you don't meet these criteria, you may not be a candidate for this procedure. I met the first two, but failed the third because four of my coronary arteries were blocked.

A report published by the American College of Cardiology in early 1991 describes the procedure as being extremely safe. Even so, about 4 percent of patients have some adverse reaction to the treatment, with one of every one hundred patients failing to survive. Three to 6 percent of the patients who have angioplasty will require urgent coronary bypass surgery.

During the actual procedure, the patient is awake but sedated, just as in the course of catheterization. The surgeon makes a small hole in the patient's right arm or groin. The balloon-tipped catheter is inserted and threaded into the blocked coronary artery. When the center of the balloon reaches the narrowest point of the blockage, the balloon is inflated for twenty to ninety seconds, sometimes longer. After this, it is deflated and the surgeon withdraws the catheter. Next, the team members inject a dye to find out if the vessel was opened by the angioplasty. The patient is taken to a recovery room, then a regular hospital room, and usually released after three or four days.

Stents

A new device used to unblock and keep open obstructed heart arteries made by Johnson & Johnson, the Palmaz-Schatz Balloon-Expandable Stent, was approved by the Food and Drug Administration (FDA) on August 3, 1994. Before granting their approval, the FDA reviewed the records of some two thousand men and women patients at forty-eight medical centers in North America and Europe.

You may think of the stent as a tiny metal scaffold that is put in place by a special balloon catheter, which is then withdrawn, leaving the stent behind to keep the blocked vessel open.

Stent insertion is gradually being accepted as a routine treatment for blocked coronary arteries. Dr. Donald Baim was quoted in April 1991 as saying that stents were used in about 15 percent of all the angioplasties done at Beth Israel Hospital in Boston. It seems to me that stents are worth looking into as a way to avoid bypass surgery.

Atherectomy Catheters

This procedure was perfected by Dr. Simon Stertzer, director of medical research for the San Francisco Heart Institute and one of Dr. Gruentzig's associates in devising balloon angioplasty.

Atherectomy involves placing a device much like a miniature Roto-Rooter at the end of a catheter that is introduced into the blocked coronary artery. This device is equipped with a tiny drill that rotates at very high speed (195,000 rpm) and actually cuts through the plaque. The procedure remains experimental, although Dr. Stertzer has reported doing more then three hundred atherectomies, with a success rate of 96 percent.

In 1993, the FDA approved the Simpson Atherocath as the first atherectomy device for coronary use.

Lasers

Another experimental method of treating blocked coronary arteries involves using a catheter that is tipped with a balloon and a heat-generating laser. Inflating the balloon pushes the plaque against the arterial walls. Then it is literally baked by heat from the laser. This technique was developed several years ago by Dr. Richard J. Spears (then at Beth Israel Hospital in Boston).

Lasers have also been used to repair abrupt closure of a

blood vessel, a problem that occurs after some angio-plasties.

Enhanced External Counterpulsation

An experimental procedure in 1994, enhanced external counterpulsation is a treatment for angina that employs a device that pumps blood from extremities to the heart. In a brief report at the 1992 meeting of the American College of Cardiology, researchers at the State University of New York told of a seven-week trial of counterpulsation treatment on eighteen patients. Twelve showed no blockage after treatment. All eighteen patients were pain-free after the treatment. The treatment costs about $7,000, is painless, and requires an hour a day for thirty-six days.

Experimental Procedures (As of Late 1995)

Mini Bypasses & Closed Chest CABG Surgery

The fact that there are now an estimated 11 million Americans who have advanced coronary artery disease makes for a market always looking for new ways to extend life. When it comes to surgery, most often the less time spent in the operating room, the lower is the cost and the greater are the chances for favorable outcomes.

One experimental procedure, a "mini-bypass," could replace conventional CABGs. It was discussed at the November 1995 meeting of The American Heart Association.

For this closed chest operation, mammary-artery grafts are inserted into a beating heart via small (band-aid-size) incisions in the chest.

Angioplasty or Bypass?

When Dr. John Ambrose saw that I was a comparatively healthy patient, with no history of a heart attack, he told me that he hoped I could avoid bypass surgery with angioplasty. When he did the angiography, however, it became clear that I had four blocked coronary arteries, with two of the blockages not accessible to the balloon. This made a bypass virtually inevitable, in my case. There is no question, however, that when there is a choice, angioplasty is preferable to CABG surgery. Angioplasty is much easier on the patient because it does not involve opening the chest, takes a lot less time (about two hours compared with four to six hours for a bypass), is associated with a shorter hospital stay and faster recovery, and costs on the average about one-third the cost of a coronary bypass. As Alix Kerr, a reporter for *Physician's Weekly*, wrote early in 1993, "From 1983 to 1990, [the] already common CABG doubled while PTCA grew ninefold. At about $12,000 a patient, Dr. Eric Topol, cardiology chair of the Cleveland Clinic, estimates that it cost taxpayers $5 billion a year for this procedure."

Kerr reported in another *Physician's Weekly* article reporting on 15 years' experience with angioplasty, that the British Randomized Intervention Treatment of Angina trial showed that "510 PTCA patients followed for two and a half years were almost four times as likely to need angiography or interventions for recurrent angina as 501 CABG patients. CABG patients led to longer recovery . . . either was superior in averting MI (myocardial infarction) or mortality."

Complications of Angioplasty

All cardiac catheterization procedures are associated with some risk of complications, ranging from bleeding and infection to problems associated with the insertion of the catheter. In addition to these, angioplasty is associated with some specific problems. These include increased risk of obstruction in the coronary arteries and puncture of the coronary vessels from the insertion of the wire used to guide the balloon catheter.

The incidence of those complications is disputed. Approximately 35 percent of angioplasties are followed by restenosis, according to Dr. Fred Loop, a surgeon who spoke in early 1993 at a symposium to celebrate the fifteenth anniversary of the first CABG (done in Cleveland by Dr. René Favaloro of Argentina). Other cardiologists at the meeting disagreed, as Alix Kerr reported in *Physician's Weekly.*

Restenosis can occur in the course of balloon angioplasty immediately afterwards or several weeks or many months later. It is usually detected when the patient reports the return of angina. Only a repeat angiogram can confirm the diagnosis.

However, given the choice of living with a blocked coronary artery and angioplasty, most of us would doubtless decide that angioplasty is well worth the risk. Shopping around for the best people to do the procedure is like choosing a bypass surgeon: look for an experienced team operating in a hospital with a good rate of success. If complications occur, a second PTCA is frequently recommended and is often successful. If angioplasty does fail, bypass surgery is most often the next choice. The fact that many angioplasties are ordered without a stress test (as many as two-thirds) makes me think that, if your cardiologist recommends PTCA without a stress test, there is a good reason to seek a second opinion.

To repeat, it is also a good idea to find a cardiologist who works in a hospital that does two hundred or more PTCAs a year. The individual cardiologist should do at least seventy-five a year.

9

What You Need to Know Just before You Undergo Coronary Artery Bypass Graft Surgery

You have been scheduled for an elective coronary artery bypass graft (CABG). This means you chose to undergo this surgery instead of trying to treat your angina with medications and were not regarded as a suitable candidate for angioplasty. Let us assume that you have not had a heart attack and did not need an emergency bypass as a result of cardiac catheterization.

I further assume that, like myself, with the help of your cardiologist, you have selected a surgeon and have checked his or her credentials (see pages 56–57 on how to do this). You also have checked out the hospital where the surgery is to take place. You feel comfortable with your decision; you feel that you are in the best of all possible hands.

You have contacted your insurance company and know exactly what they will and will not pay for. You have also made all necessary arrangements to pay whatever your insurance company will not cover.

The odds that you will survive the bypass operation without suffering any serious long-term side effects are very, very good—especially if you have chosen a surgeon who does a lot of bypasses and a hospital where CABGs are routine.

Getting Your Life in Order before Your CABG

My editor felt the section that follows is much too detailed. I disagreed and left this information in, believing that the more you know about what you can do before such a life-threatening procedure as CABG, the less anxiety you will experience. I believe that "organizing" your CABG will give you more control over what happens to you and that, as a result, you are likely to worry less and recover faster than if you were merely another passive victim of the fate that brought you to the operating table. What I intend to do is to take you through some of the actions I took when I had scheduled my CABG, hoping that you will find my experience of some help.

My first move when I knew I was going to have a bypass was to telephone my Blue Cross/Blue Shield hospitalization company. Next, I called my managed care company (Provident Mutual Life) for information about the limits of payment for my operation.

At Provident Mutual, I was told (after reciting my identification number) that, under my plan, I was responsible for 20 percent of the first $2,000 ($400), after which Provident Mutual would pay for everything else, including physicians' fees and presurgical and surgical costs. I asked if this included consultations with cardiologists, outpatient exercise tests, and the fees of anesthesiologists and surgeons. I was assured that my plan would cover these and was told that all physicians should send their bills directly to the plan office in Wallingford, Connecticut. At Blue Cross/Blue Shield, I was informed that all my hospital charges would be covered. I was then asked to call another 800 number for my "managed care" authorization to obtain a case number.

Getting that case number was not a one-step process. I

was asked to supply the name and phone number of the cardiologist who had recommended the operation so that he could be contacted by a nurse. I was also told that I must have a second opinion before I could get a case number.

When I made the calls to check in with my managed care provider, it was Friday. (The operation took place the next Monday.) My cardiologist called on Saturday to let me know he had talked to the managed care provider's nurse and had given her the information she asked for. I never spoke to anybody else connected with either insurance company and was operated on four days after I made the calls described in the preceding paragraphs. End of story. I have receipts for a total of about $95,000 paid out by Blue Cross/Blue Shield and Provident Mutual. Not a single call or letter was ever transmitted to verify any charge. What this indicates is that the system could use some checks and balances. For example, why were my charges $95,000 when the average cost in New York City is about $20,000? No one asked that question, as far as I can see.

All we had to pay for were three days of private-duty nursing and about ten days' rental for my TV set. Carole felt the nurses were necessary when I was taken from the coronary care unit to a private room. (This contained a second bed; however, it was not occupied during my stay, so I paid the double-room rate.)

Finally, I called my neighbor in Canaan, Charlie, who was then in an Atlanta hospital recuperating from *his* four-vessel CABG, in order to get a firsthand report on just what to expect. He was completely at ease and told me he had had no pain at any time during the surgery nor during the next three days. (I had called on the third day.) He also expected to be back home in Canaan within a few more days, and said he would be seeing me. "You'll be making all those telephone calls in ten days," said Charlie. "No problem!"

He was almost right. Five to seven days is the usual time

period for hospitalization after a four-vessel CABG. My own stay lasted thirteen days because of unexpected complications.

That same weekend, I made sure that Carole knew where to find all my personal papers, including my will, insurance records, lawyers' names, bank records, financial records, and so on. I also made sure that letters I had written to my wife and children would be found easily, just in case I was the one in a hundred who would not come home from the hospital. I also spent several hours calling other friends who had recovered from the same operation I was to have two days later. No one tried to dissuade me. No one said he or she was sorry about having had a CABG. All had said that their quality of life had improved dramatically. Needless to say, I felt a lot better after having made those calls.

I did not have the time to arrange for a deposit of my blood in the hospital's blood bank. I knew that I would probably need replacement blood after I was put on the heart-lung machine. I found out later I was given several units of blood from the Mount Sinai Blood Bank. Obviously none was mine. I did worry for sometime that there was a chance that it was blood from one or more donors who carried the human immunodeficiency virus (HIV). No matter how much I was reassured, I did worry, enough to ask for an HIV test a few months after my surgery. Fortunately the test results were negative.

The best way to avoid this worry is for a patient who knows she or he is to undergo bypass surgery to arrange for an autologous blood donation prior to the surgery. I suggest you ask your cardiologist if a donation is possible and if it can be arranged.

I spent the last day before I entered the hospital alone with Carole. We spoke very little. I remember spending much of the day lost in thought, sitting in the backyard of our old farmhouse.

The next day, a Sunday in early July 1989, I got up to prepare for my train trip to New York City. The surgeon's scheduler had instructed me to be admitted to the hospital around 7:00 P.M. for my operation on Monday morning.

Just before driving to the station, I did something which I now realize was pretty stupid in tempting and defying fate. (I am sharing this information to give you some insight into the personality of this person who is giving you advice.) I had found some time on Saturday to buy a new blue, 18-speed, lightweight Ross touring bike—sort of as a talisman which I felt would ensure I would be coming back to ride it. I put that bike in the barn, carefully covered by its plastic bag.

Just before leaving for the station, I went to the barn to make sure everything had been put away properly. I saw the bike. Then and there, I decided to take a short ride. The ride was not short and proved to be an incredible experience. Up and down several very steep hills I went for about an hour and a half, sweating and huffing and puffing away—without any chest pain. That ride was the first strenuous exercise I had had in about two months ever since a slight discomfort subjected me to the scrutiny of three cardiologists, two exercise tests, an angiogram, and whatever else the coming days would bring.

Why I did not suffer a heart attack as a result of that bike ride I will never know. It was only months later, after I had recovered completely, that I told Dr. Simon Dack. He said simply (sounding and looking horrified) that it was probably my highly developed collateral circulation that had saved me from having a heart attack, or worse. I hope reading about this joyride will prevent you from taking such a reckless chance with your life.

Admission to the Hospital

Getting admitted to the hospital was easy and somewhat amusing. The entire procedure took about an hour. Mount Sinai in New York is a CABG "factory," which made my case just one among hundreds done there each year. My managed care health provider identification card helped to satisfy the admitting officer about answers to the first few questions. (I believe that, without proof that the hospital would be paid, I would never have been admitted.) The amusing incident involved payment in advance for a TV in my room (see page 26).

With the formalities taken care of, I was taken to my room with my whole family in tow. My blood chemistry test records were already in the hospital's computer, as I had had the angiogram only days before. The hospital also had my ECG and film and video records of my blocked arteries.

After going for a routine chest X-ray, we returned to the room and I was told to hand Carole my personal possessions, including my wristwatch and my wedding ring. As I did this, it dawned on me that the hospital did not want to be held responsible for these personal possessions. I knew then, perhaps for the first time, that I might not need them again. This was very upsetting and precipitated my first attack of anxiety since the diagnosis of coronary artery disease. Reviewing that experience makes me think that the hospital's authorities could have been a little less business-like and a lot more humane simply by telling me what one of my friends told me later, that rings and watches frequently disappear in even the best hospital. Some of my other thoughts at the time have been described in the Introduction.

10

The Bypass Operation

(Caution: This chapter describes bypass surgery in graphic detail. You may want to skip it.)

Because some of you may want to know exactly how the surgical team performs a CABG, I will describe in some detail what happened to me after I was anesthetized. Not all surgeons do everything the same way, however; therefore, parts of my account may not match exactly what your surgeon will do for your operation. You can ask him or her to explain what will be done to you and compare what you hear to what you read here. I asked for the information before I had the surgery.

One of my first questions after I agreed to my CABG was about postsurgical pain. You may recall from the introduction that I have no memory of any pain from the moment I was given an injection in my room to the time I woke up in the coronary intensive care unit after my six-hour, four-vessel bypass operation.

Today, five years later, the only visible reminders of my CABG are two scars. One is a very thin, almost invisible fourteen-inch scar on my chest that begins about ten inches below my chin and ends about six inches above my navel. The other is a line, not as thin, that starts on my right thigh just above the knee and extends for twelve inches towards the crotch.

On the Sunday evening before my surgery, I took a shower and scrubbed myself with antibacterial soap. I was

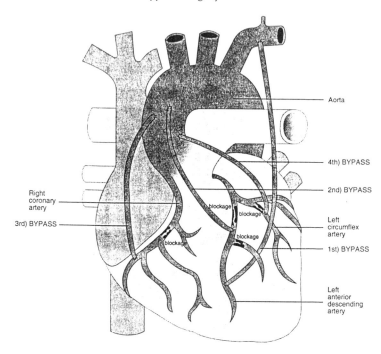

Ted's 4 vessel CABG 7/17/89

given a light meal and went to sleep about 10 P.M., with the help of a sedative.

A nurse awakened me early Monday morning and gave me a Valium injection. I was placed on a gurney and wheeled down the hall to an elevator that took me to the operating room. I had asked to be scheduled as the first patient that day. My reason for wanting to be number one: I thought the surgery team would be less likely to be tired if I started their day than if I were the third patient to be operated on that day.

Here is what I have been told happens to a patient who is prepared as I was with an injection that sedates the patient before he or she enters the operating room. The patient is washed again with antibacterial soap. All the hair from the chest area, both legs, and the pubic area is shaved. (For me, one of the few postsurgical discomforts I experienced was itching as the hair grew back.) The first of seven needles, each connected to a thin tube, is placed in a vein on the patient's right arm and taped in place, for intravenous injections. The first injections will be of anesthetics, followed by other solutions in the course of surgery, and afterwards. Another needle is inserted into an artery on the left wrist. This will be used to administer the blood-thinner, heparin, in order to prevent clotting; it will also be connected to a device that measures blood pressure. A third needle and tube is inserted into the vein near the left elbow and threaded into a vein near the heart. This will enable the anesthesiologist to deliver medication directly into the heart if that proves necessary either during or after the operation. It will also be connected to a device that measures blood pressure.

A rubber mask is fitted over the nose and mouth of the still-conscious but sedated patient. A tube attached to this mask will be used to deliver an anesthetic, usually preceded by oxygen and nitrous oxide. After this further sedation, a laryngoscope is passed down the patient's throat, past the vocal cords, providing a straight line for the insertion of an endotracheal tube. This tube will be the conduit through which the anesthesiologist will administer a muscle relaxant, as well as various anesthetic gases, to make sure there is no body movement during the operation. The same tube will be used to give the patient oxygen and other gases to neutralize the anesthetic and to awaken the patient when the operation is over.

When the patient is asleep, surgical team members insert a catheter into the bladder to remove urine and place a device for taking body temperature in the rectum. A tube is inserted in the nose and threaded down the throat to the stomach to permit the venting of fluids and gases during surgery. Another needle connected to a tube is inserted in the jugular vein.

As the name of the procedure suggests, a bypass operation involves constructing a pathway for blood from the aorta to some point beyond where the coronary artery is blocked. The material for the conduit is usually a segment of a blood vessel in some other part of the patient's body. In my case, one of the surgeons removed a vein from my right leg to construct two of the four bypasses. (The material for the other two bypasses came from mammary arteries in my chest.)

By now, the patient's chest is open and held open by clamps to permit easy access to the still-beating heart, which is now visible. The patient's entire body has been cooled from its normal ninety-eight-plus–degree temperature to about thirty-six degrees, just a little above freezing. There is good reason for this: the low temperature slows bodily reactions, so that organs and tissues need less oxygen.

It is time for the surgeon to connect the patient to the heart-lung machine. This is done by means of tubes which have been prepared by another member of the team. The heart is stopped, and the heart-lung machine takes over. As soon as the heart has ceased moving, the surgeon starts to make the bypasses, working as rapidly as possible to minimize the amount of time the patient remains on the heart-lung machine. Each of the grafts, made from a previously "harvested" blood vessel, is carefully sewn into place with tiny stitches. The grafts are closely watched for leaks and to make sure they are "patent" (wide open) before the heart-lung machine is turned off and the patient's heart is allowed to start again.

The operation is almost finished. The surgeon attaches thin wires for an external pacemaker to the heart (to correct any irregular heartbeats which may occur after the heart-lung machine is turned off.) This pacemaker will stay with the patient in the coronary intensive care unit until the surgeon is satisfied that it is no longer needed.

As the patient's heartbeat slowly returns to normal, with warmer blood circulating in his or her blood vessels, the surgeon closes the chest and the patient is taken to the recovery room. This may be three, four, or more hours from the time he or she was brought into the operating room. Actual time on the heart-lung machine can vary from less than an hour to several hours. Recovery from the bypass surgery now begins.

11

Waking Up in the Cardiac
Intensive Care Unit

One of the reasons I wrote this book was to provide some landmarks along the way for people enroute to a CABG. Having had the experience, I hope to give you the benefit of a warning where I had had little. I hope that information given in advance about an experience which I found traumatic will eliminate some of the surprise (or, shall I say, shock?). Therefore, I hope that you will read this chapter before you are taken to the operating room.

For one thing, it may help you avoid the panic that I experienced. Even though my friend Dick Morris warned me that I would not be able to speak when I woke up after surgery, I did not remember what he said when I woke up. So, I say, think about not being able to talk before you get that injection in your room. Think hard, so it will be imprinted into your consciousness. I wish it had been my last conscious thought—because if I had remembered that when I emerged from the anesthesia, I would have avoided real panic. Only I didn't. So I will tell you what happened to me, but before I recount my experiences, let's discuss what is likely to be your experience.

After your CABG is finished, you will be taken to a Cardiac Intensive Care Unit (CICU). This is a brightly lit room where you will arrive, still unconscious, stretched out on a bed with almost every one of your vital functions monitored or controlled, with the appropriate organ connected to a device or a tube. One device will breathe for you, one will remove your urine, one will monitor your pulse, and one will measure the electrical activity of your heart.

In order for the breathing unit to work, you will have a tube that is inserted down your throat through your mouth. That tube, made of a firm rubberlike material, is connected to a respirator, a device that takes in room air and can be set to "take a breath" every few seconds. Because the end of that tube is beyond your vocal cords, in order to facilitate direct access to your lungs, you will not be able to talk until it is removed.

Tubes have been inserted into your chest to remove the fluid that accumulates there after surgery. A tube was inserted into your urethra in the operating room to drain your urine; it is still in place. Another small tube, leading to a needle that has been inserted into a vein in your hand or arm, will be used to supply you with (at first) distilled water containing a little salt and liquid antibiotics (if necessary). One or both of your legs will be immobilized if that is where the vessels for the bypass graft or grafts came from. You will be linked to sensors that are connected to monitors that are hooked up to warning buzzers; the buzzers go off if there is any change from the "normal" values set by the nurses. If, for example, your heart starts to beat faster or slower for some reason, a buzzer will go off at the nursing station, where someone is constantly monitoring each patient in every bed. (All that technology and staffing is expensive, which is why one day in the CICU can cost $2,000 or more.)

Get the picture? A tube down your throat and tubes in both hands which are strapped down to a board, as are one or both legs. Thus, you are almost completely immobilized, unable to talk or even move, lying in a bed in a brightly lit and usually very noisy room, with nurses and doctors coming and going all the time.

This is the reality to which you will return following surgery, from what was, for me, a dreamless sleep. Chances are excellent you will return to consciousness, and ease into wakefulness, ever so slowly, as the anesthetics wear off.

With me, it was a gradual move into what I recognized as being alive. There was no real thought, just a life feeling. It was not that much different from the way I felt today when I woke up, just different in a matter of degree. Today, I literally woke up in an instant from a dream, but I knew where I was. My first thought was, It's Sunday and, with the sun streaming into the room, it's a good day to go to the street fair celebrating the start of the apple harvest. Today I felt good. That day, when I awoke in the CICU, I remember that some time passed before I knew "thought." I remember that the existence of me in that time and place sort of eased into consciousness. I did not know who I was, where I was, or what had happened to me. I do remember that sound and light came together with me and my being at the same time.

Ever so slowly, I started to realize that I was incredibly thirsty and my lips were very dry. That was my first feeling. Not until later did I find out that a day and a half had passed since that Monday morning when I was given an injection in my room. When I awoke, I did not think at all. I was just very, very, thirsty.

Also, I realized that I couldn't talk. Slowly realization came that I was in the room I knew to be the CICU at Mount Sinai Hospital. I opened my eyes and saw the room come slowly into focus. At the foot of my bed, not more than a few feet from my parched lips and looking at me, was a slight figure dressed in blue. He was looking at me.

I needed to inform him that my lips were dry and that I was thirsty, but I couldn't talk. I couldn't move anything except one leg. I moved that leg in a slight beat to attract his attention. He walked over to me, leaned close to my face, and as I try to remember the exact words three years later, I think he said, "There is no reason for you to beat your leg against the bed."

I couldn't believe it! He did not tell me why I couldn't talk. He did not ask if I was thirsty. He did nothing but look at me and say, "We are in charge here. You can do nothing," and walked away.

I must have gone back to sleep, for the next awareness I had was of later that day. I have been told it was evening when I awoke to see the faces of my family. It was then, hours after first returning to consciousness, that I remembered what my friend, Dick Morris, told me a few days before I went into the hospital: "The operation. The recovery. Not to worry. You won't feel any pain, but when you first wake up it may be a bit of a shocker that you won't be able to talk because they will still have you on a ventilator to assist your breathing. The tubes will be down your throat so you won't be able to talk."

If only I had remembered, I might have been spared the shock of not being able to speak, of being unable to ask for water. There is a strong likelihood that I did not need water, but I thought I did—and the panic of being unable to speak is still very much in my memory. Even though five years have passed, I still dream about it. Writing about it now I still feel the same sense of panic.

Days in the CICU will run together. You may spend two days there or maybe three before being sent to a step-down unit. My stint in the CICU lasted three days.

There were four of us in that step-down unit room, each of us with chest sensors connected to three monitors. None of us had catheters in place, none of us was on any critical list, but all of us remained under observation by nurses at a central observation station who watched TV monitors day and night to spot any changes in vital functions. A change would set off an alarm that there was a problem requiring immediate attention.

When your condition is judged stable enough, you go back to your room. Three to five days later, most patients are sent home to continue their recovery.

12

Your Rights and Responsibilities

Your hospital stay is likely to be a lot more pleasant, possibly less painful and followed by a faster recovery, if you know your rights and responsibilities. As strange as this may sound, it is true. Let me explain. I can assure you that asserting yourself in a reasonable and nonthreatening way early in the hospitalization process is likely to get you staff attention. They will start thinking of you as a person, not just another number. I also think it is reasonable to assume that an informed patient is bound to be a patient the staff of a hospital would expect to be more cooperative.

Your Rights as a Patient

The following list of patients' rights is often put on a chart easily seen in most admission offices or printed in a booklet given to every patient. Every hospitalized patient is required to receive such information. I would ask the person who admits you about it. Perhaps you should get a copy before you are admitted to see what your rights are well before you may need to know.

A hospitalized patient in New York State has the right, consistent with law, to:

1. Understand and use these rights. If, for any reason, you do not understand or you need help, the hospital must provide assistance, including an interpreter.

2. Receive treatment without discrimination as to race, color, religion, sex, national origin, disability, sexual orientation, or source of payment.
3. Receive considerate and respectful care in a clean and safe environment, free of unnecessary restraints.
4. Receive emergency care if you need it.
5. Be informed of the name and position of the doctor who will be in charge of your care in the hospital.
6. Know the names, positions, and functions of any hospital staff involved in your care and refuse their treatment, examination, or observation.
7. A no-smoking room.
8. Receive complete information about your diagnosis, treatment, and prognosis.
9. Receive all the information that you need to give informed consent for any proposed procedure or treatment. This information shall include the possible risks and benefits of the procedure or treatment.
10. Receive all the information you need to give informed consent for an order not to resuscitate. You also have the right to designate an individual to give this consent for you if you are too ill to do so. If you would like additional information, please ask for a copy of the pamphlet, "Do Not Resuscitate Orders —A Guide for Patients and Families."
11. Refuse treatment and be told what effect this may have on your health.
12. Refuse to take part in research. In deciding whether to participate, you have the right to a full explanation.
13. Privacy while in the hospital and confidentiality of all information and records regarding your care.
14. Participate in all decisions about your treatment and discharge from the hospital. The hospital must provide you with a written discharge plan and written description of how you can appeal your discharge.
15. Review your medical records without charge and obtain a copy of your medical records for which the hospital can charge a reasonable fee. You cannot be

denied a copy solely because you cannot afford to pay.

16. Receive an itemized bill and explanation of all charges.

17. Complain, without fear of reprisals, about the care and services you are receiving, and to have the hospital respond to you and, if you request it, to receive a written response. If you are not satisfied with the hospital's response, you can complain to the New York State Health Department. The hospital must provide you with the health department's telephone number.

Your Responsibilities as a Patient

When you decide to have a CABG, you should know that, as a patient, you have certain and (at least in the state of New York) well-defined responsibilities. Accepting these responsibilities will make it likely that you will get better and more considerate care. Your main job as a patient is to do what you can to recover from the surgery with as few problems as possible. Knowing your rights may help this process, but it will not ensure it. Taking responsibility for your care will.

If you learn how the hospital system works and accept your responsibilities, chances are very good the staff will go out of their way to make your recovery as fast and as painless as they can. If, on the other hand, you become "that SOB in room 153," you may count on being the first patient awakened when the morning shift begins and the last patient to get a painkiller when the orders call for one.

As a hospitalized patient in New York State for example, you are responsible:

1. For following the hospital's rules and regulations.

2. For providing, to the best of your ability, accurate and complete details about your past illnesses and

present condition. You are responsible for telling your doctor or other hospital personnel whether you have been hospitalized in the past, what for, and what medicine or other medications you are now taking or you have with you.

3. For telling your doctor if there is a change in your condition or if problems arise in your treatment.
4. For telling the doctor or nurse if you do not understand your treatment or if you do not understand what you are expected to do.
5. For following the advice and instructions of the doctors, nurses, and other hospital personnel concerning your care.
6. For the consequences if you refuse treatment or do not follow instructions.
7. For paying your bill promptly and telling the hospital if you cannot pay the bill. If you are not paying your own bill, you are responsible for telling the hospital who will pay it.
8. For being courteous to the hospital staff and other patients and for helping keep the noise and number of visitors to reasonable levels. You may not damage or remove hospital property of other patients.
9. For honoring the 11 A.M. checkout time on the day of your discharge from the hospital.

In New York City, hospitalized patients are responsible for complying with the city ordinance which prohibits smoking when hospitalized.

13

Diet

There is no question that, as far as most of us are concerned, what we eat can have a profound effect on our coronary arteries. When we eat food with a high fat content we are assured of increasing our intake of cholesterol. It is a waxy fatlike substance (lipid) that is vital to life. There are two kinds of cholesterol: dietary and blood cholesterol. Dietary cholesterol is only found in animal products like milk and meat. Blood cholesterol is produced by our bodies. To be carried in the body, cholesterol is coated by proteins called apoproteins. Once coated, they are called lipoproteins. Lipoproteins carry cholesterol and another blood lipid, triglycerides. There are several kinds of lipoproteins: low-density lipoproteins (LDL), high-density lipoproteins (HDL), and very-low-density lipoproteins (VLDL).

Because the LDL carry cholesterol, they are called the "bad" cholesterol. When this cholesterol is deposited in the walls of arteries, lumps or "plaque" is formed. This process, atherosclerosis, clogs the artery, and this blockage, which reduces the amount of oxygen-carrying blood that gets to your heart, causes the pain of angina. The HDL pick up cholesterol and, therefore, are called the "good" cholesterol.

By measuring cholesterol, HDL as well as LDL, physicians can determine if your blood lipids are within normal limits.

The higher the total cholesterol, the lower the HDL, and the higher the risk of cardiovascular disease.

The landmark Framingham Heart Study showed that, before they reach age 65, one-third of all women and men develop one or more forms of cardiovascular disease. About 50 percent of these will die of atherosclerotic disease. High cholesterol is a sign of atherosclerosis. By reducing cholesterol, you take a major step in preventing coronary disease. Very few people with a total cholesterol of 150 mg/dl have atherosclerotic disease.

The purpose of this section is to introduce you to what a postbypass patient should know about diet—and how what you eat may play a role in the rest of your life. If you had bypass surgery due to angina, you have to reduce your total cholesterol level if you want to avoid a second encounter with a surgeon. To relearn how to eat, you can take several routes. First, you can ask your cardiologist for guidance. Mine gave me a very short lecture when I visited him a few weeks after my operation.

"Your surgery was not a cure for your coronary artery disease. It just gave you a new bit of plumbing," Dr. Simon Dack told me. "If you want to avoid yet another experience with the surgeon, you have to change your lifestyle. First and foremost, you need to control what you eat. Add exercise to that new diet and, hopefully, a way to reduce daily stress. If you do these three things, the chances are good that you won't be back in the operating room for several years, perhaps never.

"The average reduction of anginal pain from bypass surgery lasts five to seven years. That's *average*. It depends on you whether or not you beat that average. So keep your fat consumption to a minimum, your weight [for a 5'11" man] to about 165, and get involved in an exercise program within three or four months after you have had a postbypass stress test to set your limits." My weight was close to 190 pounds at the time, so I was being assigned to get rid of quite a few pounds!

There is no doubt in my mind that most office-bound city dwellers who are busy day and night in an environment filled with restaurants would benefit greatly from a session or two with a nutritionist. To get this kind of expert advice, I suggest you ask your cardiologist to refer you to a one.

In my own case, there was nothing wrong with my appetite when I came home from the hospital. I began to reduce my fat intake immediately. I also consulted the nutritionist at the health club that I joined. I knew it would be some months before I was ready to start an organized exercise program, but I wanted to begin my new life, with my new plumbing, on a positive note.

I also started to read up on possible lifestyle changes, and was soon comparing the pros and cons of several well-documented approaches, each of which has a long list of ardent supporters. My research encompassed the programs (which included diet) advocated by Nathan (and now Robert) Pritikin and Dr. Dean Ornish.

Taking full advantage of either of these requires the postbypass patient to make a complete commitment. The Pritikin and Ornish methods are each very much like a religion. They are effective only if adherence is total. My problem with them was not that I didn't believe in them, just that I couldn't make the commitment. Maybe you can. If you are like me and unable to follow their recommendations, I hope that (like me) you will do the next best thing: plan your own route from their position (10 percent of total calories from fat) to something more within your capability.

There is no question that someone who is sufficiently motivated and disciplined can select and follow, with a dietitian's help, a diet in which 10 percent of the calories are derived from fat. I believe that my present diet has close to 15 percent of calories from fat. Compared with 260 mg/dl before my bypass operation, my total cholesterol level is now 180 mg/dl with the aid of one daily tablet of a cholesterol-lowering drug (Pravachol, in my case), and about forty minutes of daily exercise. As far as stress reduction is concerned, I am a complete, or almost complete, failure. In a few years, we will see how all this works out.

The current theory on the relationship between diet and lipid abnormalities that lead to coronary artery disease marked by atherosclerosis is that there are at least two basic causal disorders. One is when the LDL ("bad" cholesterol) are elevated, the other is when triglycerides rise with low HDL ("good" cholesterol). Diabetics who suffer from heart disease are known to be in that group. So if you can reduce your cholesterol with diet alone, or with diet and exercise, and as a last resort with cholesterol-lowering drugs, as well as keep your LDL low and your HDL high, you stand a good chance of reducing your risk of coronary artery disease.

But life is not so simple. In mid-1994, several articles appeared reporting on a study by Matthew Muldoon, from the University of Pittsburgh, and another study by Jay Kaplan, at Bowman Gray Medical School, that caused quite a furor. Both studies showed no net benefit for cholesterol-lowering. The Muldoon work reported that the patients they studied who were given drugs or special diets were more likely to die of violence, trauma, suicide, and accidents compared to untreated people. The Kaplan study (on monkeys) showed that monkeys that were fed a low-cholesterol diet became more violent than those that ate high-fat foods.

Then, surprise, Dr. Mark Erickson, a psychiatrist at the University of California at San Francisco, reported that monkeys are not people! He said perhaps their violence resulting from low-cholesterol diets was due to a genetic-conditioned response to less food so that aggressive (read violent) Kaplan monkeys survived over less aggressive monkeys. Erickson also said that human studies, such as Muldoon's, could be related to the fact that aggressive people have lower levels of serotonin thus perhaps lowering cholesterol may lead to lower levels of prolactin, which may lead to more victims, not fewer perpetrators. (More prolactin, less aggressive more likely to be a victim)

Then, in July of 1994, the fatty acid theory was published in *Circulation*, the official journal of the American Heart Association. This study, by Dr. Harold N. Hodis and his colleagues, concluded that it was the fatty acids (triglycerides) that contribute to the formation of plaque, or lesions, that block blood vessels and cause coronary artery disease.

What to do? As far as I can see, regardless of what causes the development of plaque, lowering your consumption of fat reduces cholesterol—and that makes sense. To avoid a second session with a surgeon, I keep my fat consumption down, try to exercise every day for about an hour, and take a cholesterol-lowering drug.

Pritikin

When medical historians write the history of diet as a method of cholesterol control, the name of Nathan Pritikin will have to be high on the list of those who made an important contribution to reducing the number of deaths from coronary artery disease. Pritikin was not a physician, not even a dietitian or member of any health team. He was simply a victim of coronary artery disease whose physician warned him he would die unless he went on a diet and agreed to take several drugs. He published the results of his self-taught program, which consisted of a diet that reduced the consumption of fat and salt, and exercise in 1949 as *The Pritikin Program for Diet and Exercise*, Gosset and Dunlap, New York.

The New Pritikin Program: The Easy and Delicious Way to Shed Fat, Lower Your Cholesterol and Stay Fit was published in 1991 by Nathan Pritikin's son, Robert. This easy-to-read book describes what has become an internationally renowned multimillion-dollar business. Its success is based on Nathan Pritikin's discovery that elimination of excess fat, cholesterol, and salt (which the Pritikins consider poisons) can prevent death from heart disease and other conditions. Many people who followed the Pritikin method have been able to lower their cholesterol levels and eliminate the use of medications.

The book also sums up other results of the Pritikins' work. You may want to read it, and if you are sufficiently impressed, you may want to take two weeks to visit one of the places (Santa Monica, California, and Miami, Florida) where the Pritikin approach is taught.

In his book, Robert Pritikin summarized some of the published results of a five-year follow-up study by R. J. Barnard and colleagues, as reported in the *Journal of Cardiac Rehabilitation* in 1983:

> Eighty-three percent of hypertensive people who entered the program on medication lowered their blood pressure to normal and left drug-free—even some participants who had been on drugs for many years.
>
> Over 50 percent of adult-onset diabetics on insulin left the program free of insulin; over 90 percent of diabetics on oral drugs left free of drugs.
>
> For many people suffering from angina, pain was greatly diminished, and 62 percent of drug-taking angina patients left the Center drug-free, while many others were able to reduce their medications.
>
> Cholesterol and triglycerides were each lowered an average of 25 percent.
>
> Overweight people lost an average of thirteen pounds during the 26-day program.
>
> Seventy percent of people suffering from claudication (blockage of the arteries of the legs) were greatly helped—even those with severe blockage and leg pains.
>
> In 1976, sixty-four people recommended for bypass surgery went through the Pritikin program instead. By

1981, 80 percent of them still had not undergone surgery.

The Pritikin approach, according to Robert Pritikin (and now based on treatment records covering 50,000 people), is "a nutritional plan in which you can eat virtually as much as you want of delicious foods without consuming dangerous amounts of cholesterol, fat, salt, and refined sugar."

The key to both the Pritikin and Ornish programs is to control the intake of dietary fat so that no more than 10 percent of total calories come from fat, 10 to 15 percent from protein, and the rest (75 to 80 percent) come mostly from complex and unrefined carbohydrates. To do this, one must follow a program and live a lifestyle that many people find far too stringent.

A friend of mine named Jim, a fifty-three-year-old singles-playing tennis buff, developed angina two years ago and decided not to have a recommended CABG. He opted for a change of lifestyle instead and has succeeded. His personal program included two stays at the Pritikin Longevity Center in Florida (early in 1993 and just recently). Jim has also become a whole-hearted believer in the Pritikin approach, to the extent of employing a Pritikin chef to spend two days in his kitchen periodically cooking and freezing hundreds of Pritikin meals.

I interviewed Jim just after he returned from his first two-week stay. He looked great, was filled with enthusiasm, and said he was convinced that Pritikin's was the way of life he would follow. His only regret was that he had not stayed for the full twenty-six day course. I repeated the interview when he returned from his second visit. He had nothing but praise again for what he went through and the way he was treated by the staff.

Jim referred himself to the Center. He told me there was no problem. "I just called and said I wanted to come down." He was there two weeks later. On his first day at the Center, he was examined in great detail by a team of physicians. Jim felt that he was given a first-class examination. With every passing day, he felt more and more part of the group. Each day, he became more adapted to the menu, which he described as full and satisfying. "I was never uncomfortably hungry," he assured me.

Jim told me that a typical day at the Center began with an early-morning exercise session which lasted about an hour. Jim enjoyed these, as well as the various classes he attended. Some of these dealt with ways to reduce stress. Some were cooking classes. Many of the participants came as couples, and as Jim observed, "It makes a lot of sense for both partners to learn the Pritikin program and stress reduction."

Jim spent a total of about $4,500 for the two weeks, including airfare from New York to Miami; $1,000 for various medical examinations; and about $3,500 for room, board, and the program. Jim said that about $700 of the costs were later reimbursed by his insurance carrier for the medical exams.

Pritikin Menu and Recipes

The basis of the Pritikin approach is nutrition plus exercise. Stress management is the third component. The key to understanding the Pritikin program is what is called "the exchange system," which allows you to select foods or "exchange" items from a well-considered list of five groups: complex carbohydrates, vegetables, fruits, dairy products, and foods that contain protein. The reason for allowing selection and exchange of foods is to prevent boredom, thus making participants more likely to follow the program for life. Because the caloric and fat content of listed foods is known, it is easy to control fat intake; there is no need to search through labels. Here is a day's menu (printed with permission from Pritikin), with selections I made for you:

Sample One-Day Pritikin Longevity Center Menu for Weight Loss

Key: Each day, eat five or more complex carbohydrates (CC), four or more vegetables (V), three or more fruits (F), only two dairy (D), and only one protein (P).

BREAKFAST (SELECT OR EXCHANGE ONE ITEM FOR EACH SELECTION)

Select ½ pita or a muffin or one piece of toast or ½ bagel. This is equal to one complex carbohydrate (CC).

½ banana or 1 orange or ½ grapefruit. Equal to one F.

Fruit du jour, ½ F exchange

Nonfat ricotta cheese (1 tbsp)

8 oz nonfat milk

3 oz nonfat yogurt

Choice of hot cereal (½ cup)

Choice of cold cereal (¾ cup)

MORNING SNACK

1 fruit

1 cup raw vegetables

½ cup vegetable soup

LUNCH

Soup 1: Spring vegetable tarragon

Soup 2: Split pea soup

Entrée: Pasta primavera (1 cup)

Vegetable du jour

Sauce: Marinara (½ cup)

Starch: Pritikin Baked Beans (½ cup)

Salad bar (1 cup)

Salads: Roma tomatoes and purple basil

Spanish noodle, cauliflower, and broccoli with mustard dressing

1 roll or ½ pita or 1 bread

AFTERNOON SNACK

Snack 1: ½ cup celery-root and baby-carrot salad, or
Snack 2: 1 cup raw vegetable medley

DINNER

Entrée 1: Turkey breast meatloaf
Entrée 2: Tamale pie (½ cup)
Sauce: Tomatillo or turkey gravy
Starch: Mashed potatoes
Vegetable du jour
Salad bar (1 cup)
1 roll
Dessert: Balsamic-marinated berries

To lose weight, emphasize soups and salads. Decrease servings of dry cereals, crackers, and bread products. Increase vegetable servings so that $CC + F = V$. Two servings of legumes or 1 serving of legumes $+ ½ P$ or $3½$ oz animal protein $= 1 P$.

Selected Pritikin Recipes

PRITIKIN BASIC DRESSING

¼ tsp red wine vinegar
¼ tsp onion powder or rice vinegar
2 tsp fresh lemon juice
1 tsp apple juice concentrate
⅛ tsp cayenne pepper
1 tsp low-sodium soy sauce
¼ tsp garlic powder
1½ tsp Dijon-style mustard
⅓ cup water
1. Place all ingredients in a jar with a tight-fitting lid. Shake vigorously for one full minute.

2. Store in refrigerator.

Makes ⅔ cup dressing. Each 2-tbsp portion contains approximately 5 calories.

ITALIAN DRESSING

Add 1½ tsp oregano, 1 tsp sweet basil, and 1 tsp tarragon, crushed with mortar and pestle, to Basic Dressing.

CUMIN DRESSING

Add ¼ tsp ground cumin to Basic Dressing.

TARRAGON DRESSING

Add 1½ tsp tarragon, crushed with mortar and pestle, to Basic Dressing.

BASIC BUTTERMILK DRESSING

4 tsp cornstarch
½ tsp dry mustard
¼ tsp garlic powder
⅛ tsp turmeric
½ cup water
1½ tsp apple juice concentrate
½ tsp low-sodium soy sauce
2 tsp cider vinegar
¼ tsp Dijon-style mustard
½ cup nonfat buttermilk
Dash cayenne pepper (optional)

1. Combine cornstarch, dry mustard, garlic powder, turmeric, and water in a pan. Stir until cornstarch is dissolved.
2. Add apple juice concentrate and soy sauce, and mix well. Place over medium heat and cook, stirring constantly until thickened.
3. Remove from heat, and add vinegar and Dijon-style mustard. Mix thoroughly.
4. Slowly add buttermilk, stirring constantly until smooth and creamy.
5. If using cayenne pepper, add it last and mix in thoroughly.

Makes 1 cup. Each 2-tbsp portion contains approximately 14 calories.

CREAMY ITALIAN DRESSING

Add ½ tsp apple juice concentrate, 2 tsp crushed oregano, ½ tsp crushed tarragon, and ½ tsp crushed basil to Basic Buttermilk Dressing.

LOUIE DRESSING

Omit cider vinegar from basic Buttermilk Dressing and substitute 1 tbsp fresh lemon juice. Add 2 tbsp tomato sauce and ½ tsp apple juice concentrate.

HORSERADISH DRESSING

Omit cider vinegar from Basic Buttermilk Dressing and substitute 1 tbsp fresh lemon juice. Add 1 tsp horseradish.

CURRY DRESSING

Omit cider vinegar from Basic Buttermilk Dressing and substitute 1 tbsp lemon juice. Add ¼ tsp curry powder.

LEMON TARRAGON DRESSING

Omit cider vinegar from Basic Buttermilk Dressing and substitute 1 tbsp fresh lemon juice. Add 2 tsp crushed tarragon.

BOSTON BAKED BEANS

4 cups cooked navy beans
2 tbsp cider vinegar
1½ cups chopped onion
1 tsp fresh ginger
1 clove garlic, minced
1 tsp dry mustard
⅔ cup tomato paste
¼ tsp ground cloves
¼ cup apple juice concentrate
⅓ tsp ground cardamom
1 tbsp low-sodium soy sauce

dash cayenne pepper
3 tbsp water
  Mix together all ingredients. Cover and bake at 350 degrees
for 1 hour. Makes 10 servings. Each ½-cup portion contains
approximately 124 calories (¼ fruit serving; 1 complex
carbohydrate serving; 1 vegetable serving).

BALSAMIC VEGETABLES

2 stalks celery cut lengthwise into strips
1 zucchini cut lengthwise into strips
1 to 2 carrots cut lengthwise into strips
Balsamic vinegar
  Steam vegetables. Sprinkle with balsamic vinegar. Serve hot.
Makes 4 servings, each containing 25 calories (approximately 1
vegetable serving).

CREAMY STIR FRY

1 cup defatted chicken stock
½ cup thinly sliced carrots
½ cup thinly sliced celery
½ cup thinly sliced zucchini
½ cup sliced green pepper
½ cup sliced mushrooms
½ tsp garlic powder
1 tsp crushed thyme
1 tsp low-sodium soy sauce
2 tsp cornstarch
⅓ cup powdered nonfat milk

1. Bring ¼ cup of the chicken stock to a boil; add carrots.
   Cook, stirring frequently, for 3 to 4 minutes. Add remaining
   vegetables and seasonings and a little more chicken stock if
   needed. Cook, stirring frequently, until the vegetables are
   crisp-tender.
2. Combine remaining chicken stock with the cornstarch and
   powdered milk. Stir until cornstarch and powdered milk are
   completely dissolved.

3. Pour cornstarch mixture into vegetables and stir until thickened. Serve immediately.

Makes 4 servings, (approximately ¼ dairy serving and ¼ vegetable serving). 55 calories each.

TORTILLA SOUP

6 cups defatted beef or chicken stock
½ cup chopped white onions
1½ cups chopped green peppers
½ cup tomato sauce
1 chopped jalapeño chili
1 clove garlic, minced
1½ cups chopped tomatoes
1 dozen corn tortillas
1 cup chopped green onions

1. Place stock in a 3-quart pan. Add white onions, ½ cup of the green pepper, tomato sauce, jalapeño, garlic and ½ cup of the tomatoes. Cook for about 15 minutes.
2. Cut tortillas into ¼-inch strips. Place on a cookie sheet and toast in a 350-degree oven for about 8 minutes until crisp.
3. To serve, place one cup of broth into a bowl with ½ cup tortilla chips. Garnish with 2 tbsp each of chopped green pepper, chopped tomato, and chopped green onion.

Makes 8 servings. Each 1-cup portion contains 105 calories (approximately 1 complex carbohydrate serving and 1 vegetable serving).

SPLIT PEA SOUP

This soup may be frozen. Why not double this recipe? You will have enough for several servings by dividing and freezing.

5 cups defatted chicken stock
1 cup split peas
Bouquet garni (2 bay leaves, ½ tsp thyme, celery leaves, and parsley sprigs).
1 clove garlic, chopped
1 small carrot chopped

1 stalk celery without leaves, chopped
1 small onion, chopped
1 leek, white part only, chopped
1 tsp thyme

1. Combine chicken stock, split peas, bouquet garni, and garlic and cook 20 minutes.
2. Add carrot, celery, onion, leek, and thyme and cook an additional 40 minutes. Remove bouquet garni. Puree. Heat thoroughly before serving.

Makes 6 servings. Each 1-cup portion contains 105 calories (approximately 1 complex carbohydrate serving and 1 vegetable serving).

CHINESE TOMATO SOUP

1 green chili, seeded, rinsed, and finely chopped
1 cup salt-free tomato sauce
15 oz can unsalted tomatoes
3 cups chicken broth or water
1 cup bok choy, cut diagonally
1 stalk celery, sliced, without leaves
1 medium white onion, thinly sliced
2 cloves garlic, minced and finely chopped
1 cup bean sprouts
½ cup chopped green onion
¼ cup cooked brown rice
1 tbsp low-sodium soy sauce
½ tsp curry powder

1. Combine chili, tomato sauce, tomatoes, broth, bok choy, celery, onion, and garlic. Cook for about 15 minutes.
2. Add bean sprouts, green onions, rice, soy sauce, and curry powder and mix thoroughly. Cook for 3 minutes and serve.

Makes 6 servings. Each 1-cup portion contains 50 calories (approximately 2 vegetable exchanges).

KIM CHEE

¼ cup rice vinegar
3 tbsp apple juice concentrate

2 tbsp fresh-grated garlic
2 tbsp grated ginger
1 tsp low-sodium soy sauce
1 tsp dried red pepper flakes
¾ cup green onion
4 cups Napa cabbage, sliced thinly

Mix all ingredients, except the Napa cabbage. Then add the cabbage to the mixed ingredients. Let sit for at least ½ hour to let flavors blend. Makes five 1-cup servings, each containing 48 calories (approximately 1 vegetable serving, and ¼ fruit serving).

MOLDED CRANBERRY SALAD

2 tbsp plus 1 tsp gelatin, unflavored
½ cup hot water
1 qt cranberry juice, unsweetened
1 cup apples, peeled and diced
9-oz jar cranberry sauce
1 cup sugar

Dissolve gelatin in hot water and stir in ¼ cup of the cranberry juice. Stir in remaining cranberry juice, mix in sugar, and refrigerate. When gelatin begins to thicken, mix in apples and cranberry sauce. Pour into 7-cup mold. Return to refrigerator until firm. Makes 14 servings, 70 calories each (approximately 1 fruit serving).

14

Exercise—Less Is More

In June 1994, a group of Helsinki researchers led by Dr. Timo Lakka published the results of a 1984–89 study of 1,453 men forty-two to sixty years old who did not have cardiovascular disease or cancer. The authors concluded that "higher levels of both leisure-time physical activity and cardiorespiratory fitness had a strong, graded, inverse association with the risk of acute myocardial infarction, supporting the idea that lower levels of physical activity and cardiorespiratory fitness are independent risk factors for coronary heart disease in men."

There is no question in my mind that physical activity can help prevent coronary artery disease. Every postbypass patient should develop and maintain a carefully planned exercise program. You will need help from at least two experts to devise that program. First, you should consult your cardiologist to find out how soon after surgery you should start exercising and how to pace yourself so you don't put too much stress on your new plumbing. Second you should consult an exercise physiologist or someone trained to help postbypass patients develop safe exercise programs.

My first postbypass exercise began when I was given a red heart-shaped pillow as I was taken from the step-down unit back to my hospital bed. The nurse who gave it to me explained that I should squeeze it regularly to help get my chest muscles back in condition. Along with the pillow came a device into which I was supposed to blow with sufficient force to make a little ball go to the top of a tube, also to help those chest muscles.

The first attempt at both squeezing and blowing hurt every muscle in my chest, but the pain was bearable enough for me to go on trying. A few minutes of every waking hour was spent squeezing the pillow and blowing on the tube device. After a few days, the pain stopped. It became easier to squeeze that pillow and a lot easier to keep that ball at the top of the tube.

About the fifth day after surgery, I was taken for my first postbypass walk. Getting from my room to the end of the corridor and back was quite a challenge! I did it, though, and every day after that victory I was taken on longer and more frequent walks and allowed to sit in a chair in my room. By the time I left the hospital, thirteen days after surgery, I was able to take ten-minute walks four or five times a day.

My second exercise regimen began the day I went home when I managed to walk about half a New York City block. That's about five hundred yards. Each day after that, with Carole's help, I lengthened the walk. A month after surgery, I was walking for thirty minutes, twice a day. Most cardiologists say that walking is the safest, easiest, and often the best exercise for almost everyone, especially the postbypass patient.

About three months after surgery, I was able to walk with no discomfort or pain. I made a two-week trip to Italy, walking every day for three or four hours, without any of the discomfort that sent me to surgery. I was bored with just walking, however, and asked my cardiologist when I could start swimming and biking again.

Dr. Simon Dack said that, before he would suggest anything more vigorous than walking, I should take an exercise stress test with a radioisotope to see if my bypass had, in fact, resulted in four new open vessels. I did as he suggested and was given a great report. All the grafts were open. There were no problems according to the cardiologist who ran me on the treadmill. "You can jog, run, swim, climb mountains—anything you want to do, but keep your heart rate at no more than about 144 beats per minute."

I was told I could exercise for as long as I wanted, up to 144 beats per minute, without any danger. In fact, the doctor who ran me on the treadmill encouraged me to do precisely that every other day for the rest of my life. And now, five years after my bypass, that is what I am still doing.

There is another way to calculate a safe range of exercise. This program comes from Dr. Siegfried Kra's book, *Coronary Bypass Surgery: Who Needs It.* You will need the help of a cardiologist or exercise physiologist or both to work out this program.

Dr. Kra recommends exercise that is equivalent to 70 percent of the maximum rate of oxygen consumption on a treadmill, measured in mets. A met is the metabolic equivalent of 3.5 milliliters of oxygen per one kilogram body weight per minute at rest. His example is a man whose maximum tolerance is 10 mets when jogging on a treadmill. This patient's exercise prescription would be to go no higher than seven mets, or 70 percent of the 10 mets— allowing him to jog at the rate of five miles per hour, to bike at 12 mph, and swim one mile in an hour. That's seventy-two lengths in an Olympic pool.

Patients recovering from a bypass should not walk faster than 3 mph for some months. Most of us will not be going any higher than 8 mets after our cardiologists consider us ready for greater stress.

Yet another system to help you decide how much exercise is enough is measured in "aerobic points." This is the system that Dr. Kenneth H. Cooper, the man who created the word "aerobics" in 1968, has established. It is described in his book, *The Aerobics Program For Total Well-Being.* Cooper has had a great impact on aerobic exercise, and many people follow his recommendations.

His system involves assigning points for a specific activity carried out for a given distance for a specific time. To achieve and maintain aerobic fitness, the Cooper goal is to record thirty-five or more points each week for the rest of your life. You can score thirty-five points by jogging nine miles a week, skiing for about six hours, or playing racquetball for four hours. Many people like the Cooper Method because it is varied enough to keep them from getting bored.

Rather than worry about mets, points, or oxygen, Dr. Kra wrote that, as far he can see, "A daily, brisk, long walk (two to three miles) can be an excellent substitute for jogging!" I agree.

Many articles and books explain how to start a regular walking program. After doing the research for this book, and after many attempts to get into an exercise program that would work for me, I believe that walking is, by far, the best physical activity for postbypass patients and almost everyone else. There is now a vast amount of literature on walking. I recommend you look into it seriously before you begin any exercise program.

The single best source of information about walking for exercise, as far as I am concerned, is in an article by James M. Rippe, M.D., and colleagues. It was printed in the *Journal of the American Medical Association* (259, no. 18 [May 13, 1988]: 2720–24). I strongly recommend that you go to a library and read it. Better still, get a photocopy from the library and make notes. Then you will have all the references you need right at home, including the titles of several books that describe how to test your physical status, or "walking readiness." Once you have the results of this self-administered test, you can devise your own walking program to help you keep fit.

The "One-Mile Walk Test" was developed by Dr. Rippe. It was adopted and, for a while, promoted by the Rockport Company, a shoe manufacturer (now owned by Reebok). Part of this promotion was a pamphlet, which included an excellent guide to help test a person's walking fitness. This guide is, unfortunately, no longer available, but studying Dr. Rippe's article will show you how to take the test and then set up your own program. Also, chapter 10 in *Prevention of Coronary Heart Disease,* edited by Drs. Ira S. and Judith K. Ockene, is an excellent source of detailed information on the benefits of exercise.

Everything I have learned indicates that a postbypass patient should exercise for an hour or so, five days a week. You should start slowly and work up to where you may be pushing a bit—but *not to where it hurts.* I believe that the no-pain, no-gain adage was created by orthopedic surgeons to help pay for what they may consider a higher standard of living.

Another excellent guide is *Walk Your Way to Fitness and Health,* by Fred A. Stutman, M.D. It was published by Ballantine, and I recommend that you get a copy as soon as you can. Every postbypass patient who is thinking about an exercise program should give serious consideration to Dr. Stutman's thoughts on the subject. He found, as part of his research, an early 1970s article in the *Journal of the American Medical Association,* whose authors had looked into the cause of death in eighteen joggers. They found there was no way to predict the runners' deaths in advance, leading Dr. Stutman to advise, "Walk, do not run." I agree. I keep meeting more and more male and female joggers who complain about sprains, strains, fractures, and other injuries. Many of them seem to be addicted to jogging. As far as I can tell, the worst cases are the marathon runners, many of whom give up all of their free time (and, some, not-so-free time) to compete.

Dr. Stutman reminds us that walking at even *moderate* speed can double your heart rate. This easy, and safe, aerobic exercise doesn't cost much, can be done anywhere, and becomes enjoyable for most people who do it. The book also includes a section entitled "How Walking May Help Reduce the Risk of Heart Attack," in which Dr.

Stutman lists the benefits of a regimen of regular walks. He writes that walking:

1. Lowers the resting heart rate
2. Promotes faster return of heart rate to normal after exercise
3. Decreases the resting blood pressure
4. Improves the efficacy and capacity of the lungs
5. Increases the blood's volume and oxygen-carrying capacity
6. Decreases circulating blood fats
7. Increases the flexibility of the blood vessels and expands the size of the arteries including the heart's own coronary arteries
8. Increases the high-density lipoproteins (HDL), which are the molecules of fat and proteins in the blood that appear to exert a protective effect against heart disease
9. Lessens the chance of blood clot formation
10. Improves the heart's maximum cardiac output (total volume of blood expelled from the heart)

If you can, read the entire book. If you are in a hurry to get started, read chapters 4, 5, 6, 7, and 8. Dr. Stutman's list of organizations that promote walking is especially worthwhile. A really dedicated walker can even learn how to get a free index of topographical maps from the U.S. Geological Survey. But don't ignore this warning: although walking is one of the safest and least strenuous forms of exercise, be sure to consult your own physician before embarking on a walking exercise program.

All of this talk about exercise may cause you to ask, why exercise at all? The answer is because it will make you feel better. Will it eliminate the need for another bypass? No one knows for certain. I had been a regular weekend jock, but after my bypass, I decided to engage in some form of exercise for an hour every day. I continue to do so and have never felt better.

I was told that I never had a heart attack despite four clogged arteries because of my regular exercise program. The reason I chose bypass surgery was because I wanted to maintain a high quality of life, including engaging in regular exercise. Later, I learned that my recovery from the four-vessel bypass operation in only six weeks was related to my body's good condition—a direct result of regular swimming, biking, and workouts.

Telling you all this is a way of introducing you to the importance of adding a regular program of exercise to your daily life after your CABG. There are all sorts of benefits. Properly performed, exercise will lead to significantly higher concentration of HDL in your blood. (See the glossary for more on high- and low-density lipoproteins.) Regular exercise will help you stay on a sensible low-fat diet. Most important of all, it will help you feel and look good. The good news is that, to enjoy the benefits of exercise, you don't have to become a jock.

Remember, all that bypass surgeon did was to put in some new plumbing; you did not receive any treatment for the coronary artery disease that caused your angina. You still have it, and you need to change your lifestyle to avoid another CABG. You need to lower your LDL level by making a real change in your diet and by reducing your consumption of fat. You need to raise your HDL level, and incorporating exercise into almost every day of the rest of your life is one way to do this.

I do not enjoy eating low-fat food. I especially miss ice cream and frequent pig-out sessions on the overstuffed corned beef and pastrami sandwiches from the Carnegie Delicatessen, a place the Michelin Guide would describe as definitely worth a detour for anyone on a gourmand's tour of Manhattan. I do enjoy my daily hour in a gym, though I prefer the way I feel after swimming a half mile as fast as I can. The two miles I walk every day (in less than thirty minutes) invigorates me.

Starting a Post-CABG Exercise Program

You need to be careful before starting on a post-CABG exercise program. Do not attempt to start a program without undergoing a complete exam by your cardiologist. He or she will probably tell you about a fitness schedule without any prompting. If this doesn't happen, you need to be tested by a physician (not by a fitness center exercise expert or trainer). The program of tests in current use at the Ochsner Medical Institution in New Orleans is one of the best I was able to find. It may help you and your cardiologist design a schedule for you. The Ochsner program for a post-CABG patient includes:

1. A graded exercise stress test
2. Blood lipid analysis: determines total cholesterol, triglycerides, low-density and high-density lipoprotein, and glucose levels
3. Body composition analysis (skin-fold measurements to determine lean body weight, fat weight, and body fat percentage)
4. Muscular strength and endurance test
5. Nutritional profile

You don't have to go through all that, but in consultation with your cardiologist, it may be a good place to start. Whatever you do, *do not* place yourself in the hands of a "trainer" or someone who claims to be trained in exercise physiology without checking their credentials. You can really hurt yourself if you don't know what is best for you.

Because I want to share what you can see is a conservative addiction, let me describe my daily schedule of exercising. I do this with some confidence that it can help you avoid a second CABG because I took a third radioisotope stress test three years after my operation. The cardiologist in charge said, "I don't know what you are doing, I really don't want to know, but keep doing it. The results of the test we just gave you tell us that you have the circulation of a man not yet 30. So, don't do anything different."

Soon after that third radioisotope stress test, and having gotten bored with my exercise routine, I asked a trainer at the gym I had been using for two years to give me a new set of exercises. I ignored the advice that the cardiologist had given me ("Don't change what you are doing"). I got into a new exercise program and did what the trainer showed me, including a ten-minute stint on the rowing machine. The result: agony—pain in the back and right leg caused by damage to the sciatic nerve. For five days, I was unable to sit for more than a few minutes; sleep was almost out of the question.

Eventually, after self-medicating failed to work, I paid a visit to my neighborhood chiropractor. Dr. Sam Sobel advised me to go to bed, to keep my legs elevated, and to stay that way for four days. He directed me to take three ibuprofen tablets three times a day.

At the end of the first day, the pain had stopped. It returned when I got up the next morning but had lessened. By the third day, there was no pain; by the fifth day, I was back in my office.

For what it's worth, here is my exercise routine: Every weekday before going to my office, I walk three blocks to a gym. I either walk for thirty minutes on a treadmill at 4.0 mph or ride a stationary bike for thirty minutes, following a program of random hills at (a moderate degree of difficulty on the bike's computer). Every other day, I lift twenty-pound weights on a schedule of about six different body-building movements. This weight routine is followed by ten minutes on a total of five or six Nautilus type machines. I don't go to the gym on weekends (it's very crowded), but

I either ride my bike for an hour and a half (halfway around Manhattan island) or swim half a mile or so in about twenty minutes at a neighborhood pool. That's it.

How Much Is Enough Exercise?

You don't have to buy a fancy outfit. You don't have to join a gym. You don't have to buy any equipment at all. Just make a modest investment in a pair of shoes. (*Consumer Reports*, May 1992, has a detailed report on tests done on thirty-two brands.) Current medical thinking is that, to maintain a good cardiovascular tone, you need only increase your heart rate for twenty minutes three times a week. You can do this by walking at about 4 mph, or strolling at 3 mph. Now, you can do that, can't you?

You can do a lot more, except that more is not necessarily better when it comes to exercise. The Wellness Center of the Ochsner Heart Institute has published an excellent short guide on cardiac rehabilitation. (You can get a copy by writing the Institute at 1512 Jefferson Highway, New Orleans, LA 70121.) This guide lists the benefits of exercise under five categories, with the potential benefits of the Center's wellness program described as

I. CARDIOVASCULAR IMPROVEMENTS

    A. Decreased resting blood pressure

    B. Decreased resting heart rate

    C. Increased maximum oxygen consumption (a measure of cardiovascular fitness)

    D. Decreased myocardial oxygen demands during submaximal exercise

II. MUSCULOSKELETAL IMPROVEMENTS

    A. Decreased body fat

    B. Increased lean body weight

    C. Improved muscle tone
    D. Improved posture
    E. Improved physique
    F. Reduction of age-related bone loss (very important for women)

III. BLOOD LIPID CHANGES

    A. Decreased levels of total cholesterol
    B. Decreased levels of triglycerides
    C. Increased HDL
    D. Decreased total cholesterol-to-HDL ratio

IV. PSYCHOLOGICAL IMPROVEMENTS

    A. Improved self-image
    B. Decreased depression
    C. Decreased anxiety
    D. Improved mental cognition and reaction time

V. MISCELLANEOUS

    A. Increased basal metabolic rate
    B. Aid in weight reduction
    C. Increased sense of well-being

Are you convinced? If not, better keep in close contact with your cardiologist. If you are planning an exercise program and think just walking will be too boring, I recommend getting help to set up a program that you will follow and enjoy because, unless you enjoy it, you won't do it. Many YMCAs, YWCAs, and even some hospitals have individual and group programs for the post–heart attack and postbypass patient. The cost for some of these may be included in your insurance package, so be sure to check that when you find one.

In their recent landmark book, *Prevention of Coronary Heart Disease* (Little, Brown, 1992), Judith and Ira Ockene, James Rippe, Ann Ward, and others discuss the benefits of exercise after bypass surgery. I like their summary. It is a lot more detailed but says in effect that a successful exercise program should

1. Be regular rather than vigorous
2. Be simple and require moderate exertion
3. Not need special facilities, equipment, or skill

Brisk walking is their ideal—and mine, too. It meets all their criteria and, even better, can be done in any weather, almost any place. Walking is inexpensive, does not require any fancy clothes, and can be done alone or with one or more equally committed friends.

15

The Answers to the Most-Often-Asked Questions about Bypass Surgery

While preparing for this part of the book, I asked cardiologists and primary care physicians in several cities around the country to keep a record of the questions most frequently asked by patients when they were told that bypass surgery was necessary. Next, I consulted experts to arrive at a consensus for answers.

Readers are invited to send me any questions that are not asked or answered here to help with the preparation of the next edition. Future patients will be grateful to you for taking the trouble. Address your questions to me in care of Ohio University Press, Athens, Ohio, 45701.

I would like to thank Drs. John Ambrose, the late Simon Dack, the late James Kaufman, Ira Ockene, Carl E. Orringer, and Harvey Wolinsky for their help in providing me with these most frequently asked questions. I am especially grateful to Dr. Ira Ockene, who not only reviewed the questions but also edited the answers I had collected from his colleagues. His and his wife's recent book, *Prevention of Coronary Heart Disease,* has also been extremely helpful. Even though it was written for physicians, I can't recommend it too highly to anyone who has had a bypass. The book might have been even more useful to you some years ago, before coronary heart disease took its toll and led you to confront the choice of surgery, but, it could still do wonders to keep you from that second surgical encounter—a goal that everyone who has had a bypass would surely agree is worthwhile.

Also, thanks to Arthur Aaron Levin, MPH, director of the Center for Medical Consumers in New York City, and publisher of *HealthFacts*, an excellent monthly newsletter.

Here are the questions and answers:

Q: Will I die as a result of the surgery?

A: It depends on several factors. The state of your health before surgery, the skill of the surgeon and her or his team, as well as the hospital where you go for the bypass. The results of over 57,000 coronary artery bypass grafts (CABGs) in thirty New York State hospitals published in the *Journal of the American Medical Association* showed that the 1992 risk of death was 2.45 percent in those hospitals. Women do face an increased risk of death following bypass surgery compared to men. In a study published by the Agency for Health Care Policy and Research for which the records of over three thousand patients were evaluated, 7.1 percent of women and 3.3 percent of men died in the hospital following CABG.

Q: Just what is a coronary bypass?

A: The bypass operation, more accurately described as a coronary artery bypass graft, involves removing one or more healthy veins from the leg or an artery from the chest wall and sewing the vessel so it bypasses the blockage in the vessels that bring blood to the heart. Thus, a CABG is a detour for blood flow. To some it is not an "open heart" operation, since the heart itself is not operated on for a bypass, only the vessels that supply the heart. More veins than arteries are used. If you define an open heart operation as one where a cardiopulmonary bypass machine is used, then a CABG *is* an open heart operation.

Q: What will arteriography tell the cardiologist?

A: Arteriography detects the presence and location of blockage of the coronary arteries that have been caused by arteriosclerosis. It also shows the functioning of the valves or vascular walls of the heart.

Q: Can I avoid bypass surgery by going to a place like Pritikin's or one run by Dr. Ornish so I won't need a bypass by just changing my lifestyle?

A: You can try. Dr. Ockene told me that if there is a high risk that a patient will have a heart attack or stroke, then surgery may be indicated. However, he feels if there is a low risk (best defined by the consulting cardiologist), it may be worth the effort and expense of investigating whether diet, exercise, and a marked change in lifestyle will further lower the risk and, thus, obviate the need for surgery. Again, the choice (to have surgery or not) must be made rationally and with the best information tion available to the most competent cardiologist. Even the doctor can be wrong, and as with everything else in life, you make your choice and take the chance.

After doing the research for this book, I believe that there are relatively few people whose need for a bypass can be avoided by substituting a radical change in lifestyle and diet. If I had been at low risk and had the time and money, I would have given the lifestyle change a try. I was at high risk, however, with four blocked arteries and was told that, unless I had a bypass, there was a clear danger of a heart attack or stroke if the operation was delayed. I was also advised that, in order to maintain my lifestyle including regular and heavy exercise, medical management would not work. So I had no choice of enrolling in a Pritikin- or Ornish-like treatment plan. I suggest you read what these authors claim is a way to avoid bypass surgery by following their lifestyle plan. Dr. Ornish's book is called *Reversing Heart Disease: The Only System Scientifically Proven to Reverse Heart Disease Without Drugs or Surgery.* That's quite a claim! According to Dr. Ornish, you could certainly avoid another bypass operation by putting yourself in his hands and following that lifestyle. (My reason for saying *another* is because most of the people who read this probably have had or soon will have bypass surgery.) If I am wrong and you are considering diet, stress reduction, and exercise as an alternative to a date with the surgeon, I would certainly think (if your cardiologist agrees) that you should take a good look at the Ornish or Pritikin method. Why not, if you have the time and are not being rushed to a bypass or medication?

Q: What are the risks of angiography, balloon angioplasty, and bypass surgery?

A: For all such procedures, epidemiologists keep records on the basis of the number of patients who are worse off (morbidity) due to the operation or test, as well as the number of patients who do not survive (mortality). Recently in the medical journal *Lancet* (344 [August 27, 1994]: 563), it was reported that patients who had bypasses had significantly lower death rates than those who were given medications instead of a bypass. That is, 26.4 percent of those who had surgery died compared to 30.5 percent of those who received medications died. It is important to know that there are several variables that can affect the results and not just the skill of the surgeon and the bypass team; your age, for example, is a factor. If you are suffering from a disease like diabetes in addition to coronary artery disease, that can also make a difference. If you are overweight, smoke two to three packs of cigarettes a day, and have hypertension, you are not going to have the same chance of surviving the operation and living several more healthy years as someone who was in excellent health before his or her need for a bypass was discovered. In addition, there is no question that, all things considered, the risk of a failure is a lot higher in a hospital where five bypasses are done each month than in a hospital in which five are done each day. In an issue of *HealthFacts,* dated April 1994, Art Levin cites a report in the *Journal of the American Med-*

ical Association (March 9, 1994) in which, in a randomized survey of three hundred U.S. hospitals that reported, the death rate from CABAGs was 25 to 30 percent higher than that found in randomized clinical trials.

Q: How soon after I am told that I need a bypass should I have the operation?

A: You may not have a choice if your cardiologist and the angiographer agree that you are in immediate need of surgery. The estimate of the risk is based on the extent of blockage or narrowing of the vessels that are major suppliers of blood to your heart. If there is relatively little blockage or narrowing, you may be given the option of trying medical treatment before surgery. On the other hand, if the angiogram shows blockage in several vessels, or what is called left main disease (defined on page 37), or you have substantial anginal pain, you will probably be asked to schedule surgery as soon as possible.

Q: How many arteries or veins are used for bypass grafts?

A: As many as are needed, depending on the number of blocked arteries and the location of the blockage. One graft will be needed to make one bypass; sometimes one graft will accomplish two bypasses (a sequential or "jump" graft). I needed four bypasses, so both of my mammary arteries and one of my leg veins were used.

Q: What other surgical and nonsurgical options are available to me besides bypass to control my angina? Why can't they just ream out or dissolve the blockage?

A: There are several options to treat blocked heart vessels other than bypass surgery. They have been done with varying degrees of success. One of these involves using a balloon (percutaneous transluminal coronary angioplasty—PTCA). A balloon is inserted to open the vessel by actually pushing the plaque up against the vessel wall so that more blood will flow through. The other methods are still experimental. One of these is atherectomy, also called the Roto-Rooter, in which an instrument is used to cut into the clogged substance and then remove it.

Lasers have also been used experimentally to open the clogged vessel.

Q: Will I have pain after my bypass?

A: If you mean anginal pain, you shouldn't have any after your operation if the bypass was effective. However, up to 40 percent of people who have bypass surgery to eliminate anginal pain have anginal pain after surgery. Is it worth the risk, expense, and days lost from work? Only you can decide.

Q: What about pain from the surgery?

A: If you wonder about the length of postsurgical pain, this depends on several factors. Your body's condition before surgery has a lot to do with it. If you were in good physical shape and did not suffer any surgical complications, chances are good that you will suffer only minor discomfort where your chest and leg (or legs) were opened for the operation. The incisions will usually heal quickly. Most often patients experience no discomfort aside from itching and stiffness of the chest and legs. I was not sore for very long after my operation, but some people who have had a bypass have told me that they were sore for a long time after coming home from the hospital. For me, actual discomfort lasted only a few weeks, while the stiffness persisted for several months; even five years after surgery, my right leg (the one from which the vein was removed) remains stiff enough to make it difficult to put my socks on when I get dressed. If you are aggressive in pursuing an exercise program, your rehabilitation will be fast.

Q: When will I be able to return to work?

A: It depends on the extent of your surgery and the shape you were in before your operation. What you do after your surgery to recondition your body is also important. If you were a couch potato before the bypass and go back to your couch after the bypass, it will take you longer to gain the energy you'll need to return to work than if you start an exercise program as soon as your physician says you can. If you were a marathon runner or any sort of a jock before bypass and want to compete again, be sure to get a thallium exercise stress test before you schedule any strenuous activity after bypass surgery.

Q: Will I still have to take medications after bypass surgery?

A: It depends on which medications you were taking, your other medical needs, and whether you change your lifestyle after surgery. For instance, if you had angina and hypertension before surgery, chances are you won't continue to take the anti-angina medications—but you will continue to need the medication for hypertension. If you don't make a major change in your diet, including eliminating fats and don't start and keep on an aggressive exercise program, you will probably have to take cholesterol-lowering medicines for the rest of your life. Your cardiologist will monitor you to make sure that your angina has been successfully treated. (Remember, all that bypass did was give you some new plumbing. It did not cure the coronary artery disease that necessitated the bypass surgery. If you don't make a major change in your lifestyle, chances are very good you will need more surgery in a few years.)

Q: Will the blockage come back?

A: There is a possibility that your newly installed vessels will become blocked. It can happen very shortly after the bypass—perhaps a week or a month later. Sometimes it happens seven to ten years later. The best estimate is that two in five, or 40 percent, of the vessels will occlude ten years after a CABG. Remember we are speaking of averages. This is not an absolute prediction that you will need another operation. There are some cases of blockage recurrence that can be treated with angioplasty (or PTCA; see page 83) in which a balloon is used to open the blood vessel, thus obviating the need for another bypass.

Q: Will I have to change my diet?

A: Probably, yes, because chances were good that your prebypass diet was high in fat.

Q: When will I be able to exercise after my bypass?

A: That depends on the extent of your surgery, your pre-surgical condition, and the amount and type of exercise you want to do. You will find that exercise is high on the list of activities your surgeon and cardiologist want you to follow. Your surgeon and cardiologist will give you a list and a guide for exercise when you have your post-surgical office visit. I was walking three weeks after my four-vessel surgery, went to Italy two months after, and was even swimming a little three months later. My full, daily, one-hour exercise in a gym was scheduled about six months later. I was given a schedule of effort (the amount of time and the heart rate I could climb to) after I had a postbypass thallium stress test. For me, at the age of sixty-three years, this meant being allowed to get my heart rate up to 144 beats per minute. See chapter 14 for more information on how to plan a rational postbypass exercise program.

Q: When will I be able to have sex after my bypass?

A: It depends on your sexual practices. For most of us, having sex means that our heart rate goes up to about 110 to 130 beats per minute. However, there have been reports that postbypass patients have an increased chance of an unexpected and unwanted cardiac problem if the sex is with an unfamiliar partner. With familiar partners, the heart rate during sex is about the same rate as that experienced while climbing a single flight of 14 stairs in ten or fifteen seconds. One way to determine if sex will cause chest pain would be to climb a flight of steps. No pain? Try having sex. Ask your cardiologist if there is any reason you should not try the stair test.

Q: Which is the best hospital to go to for a bypass?

A: One that has a surgical team that does 250 or more by-passes in a year with a success rate of 95 percent or better. It is a good idea to find out if the surgeon and hospital your cardiologist suggests come up to this mark. Ask for this information.

Q: When can I drive and travel after my bypass?

A: It all depends on what condition you were in before the bypass. If you had a heart attack, were overweight, smoked, and were sixty-five years old, it would take you longer to recover to this point than if you were in excellent condition prior to surgery. I was able to take business-related telephone calls a few days after returning from thirteen days in the hospital. I worked at home for the next four weeks, using my telephone, word processor, modem, and fax machine. I even saw a few clients who visited me during that month. About twelve weeks after my surgery, I spent two weeks in Italy on vacation. I did not try to drive until about three months after surgery.

Q: How will I know if I'm getting sick again after a bypass?

A: You will have the same old pain and discomfort or will tire easily.

Q: Can I still get a first heart attack or suffer another heart attack after a bypass?

A: Yes. But if you do, your odds for survival and fast recovery are better than if you had not had a bypass.

Q: Will I have problems because my leg veins and mammary artery were used for the bypass surgery?

A: You won't miss them. However, your leg (or legs) may show a bit of swelling (edema). My right ankle is still a bit puffy, five years after the bypass.

Q: How long will the operation take?

A: This depends on several factors which include the number of bypasses, the skill of the team, and the need to deal with unforeseen complications. Cardiologist Ira Ockene tells me that "ever since anesthesia was invented, I see no reason to rush the surgeon." In my case, four vessels were used for bypasses and about six hours elapsed from the time I was wheeled into the operating room until I was taken to the recovery room. Since you will be asleep until the next day, time will not matter.

Q: Will I have ugly scars on my chest and legs?

A: It depends on the skill of the surgeon who closes the wound made for the operation. For men, there isn't likely to be a problem. I had a fourteen-inch chest scar that is now almost invisible five years after the surgery. My right leg has also healed but was not sewn up as well as my chest, so that scar is more noticeable.

Q: How long will I be hospitalized?

A: It depends on how fast you recover from the operation. The average total time is about five days, including one day in the cardiac intensive care unit and three days in a hospital room. I was hospitalized for thirteen days because of unforeseen complications, including a second operation to repair a bleeding vessel and treatment in a step-down intensive care unit, followed by three additional days to treat a badly swollen trachea due to the trauma caused when the anesthetist inserted a second breathing tube during the second operation.

Q: What do they use for the bypasses?

A: The saphenous vein from the leg and the internal mammary arteries. Mammary arteries are the first choice because they don't occlude as often as saphenous veins. Sometimes the blockage is at a location that can't be reached with the internal mammary artery, so the vein has to be used.

Q: Why not use soft plastic tubes instead of arteries and veins?

A: As of late 1995, no plastic tube for bypass use has been approved. However early in 1993, surgeons at Abbott-Northwestern in Minneapolis for the first time used a experimental teflon device as a bypass. These are not approved by the Food and Drug Administration as of this writing.

Q: What are the odds that the bypass will successfully cure my angina?

A: About six to nine of every ten bypasses result in significant improvement or complete elimination of angina. This means the rate of failure can reach 40 percent. Failure is defined as a return of angina due to blockage (occlusion) of the bypass graft. This is one reason for the careful weighing of alternatives to bypass surgery, including medical treatment and balloon angioplasty.

Q: How long will the bypass graft or grafts work (or remain wide open)—and then what?

A: On the average, from seven to ten years. Then comes balloon angioplasty and another attempt at bypass grafting.

Q: Why can't the blockage be dissolved?

A: As of this date, there is no way to do this safely.

Q: How do I find the best surgeon for my operation?

A: You can ask the surgeon whom your cardiologist recommends to tell you his or her success-versus-failure rate for the last year. There is no consumer's guide to help you pick a surgeon. Art Levin has shown me a printout of the success-versus-failure rates for bypass surgeons in New York State. Some of these surgeons had a success rate greater than 95 percent. If you were looking just at that list and found the surgeon recommended to you was not on it or had a success rate below 95 percent, you might simply opt for another surgeon. Dr. Ockene reminded me, however, that lists of this sort can do a great disservice to surgeons who specialize in high-risk patients. Such a surgeon's success rate can be 50 percent—but those patients on whom he operated unsuccessfully might never have had a chance had they been looking for a surgeon who batted over .900!

Q: Why shouldn't I go to one of the large hospitals like the Cleveland Clinic or Debakey's unit in Houston for my bypass?

A: There is no good reason why you shouldn't go anywhere you like. There are teams that have as good a success rate in many larger, and even some smaller, hospitals. All things considered, it makes sense to go some place near where you live. My neighbor in Canaan, New York, whose family comes from Atlanta, went there to have his very successful four-vessel bypass at St. Michael's Hospital. As in most services, when it comes to choosing a surgical team, the bypass patient can shop around for the best, or even the least expensive, team. My own choice is the team with the best morbidity and mortality records that is closest to where you live, so it will be easier for your partner and family to come and visit.

Q: Will I be depressed after my CABG or suffer some brain damage as a result of my CABG?

A: Yes, you could suffer from some mood changes. I did. They lasted over a month, until I saw that my strength was returning. In 1989, *Physician's Weekly* reported that about 35 percent of CABG patients showed signs of confusion and depression immediately after surgery. After eight weeks, up to 25 percent were still affected.

Appendix

What My Husband's Bypass
Meant to Me

by Carole Klein

For me, the first moment of what was to be our terrifying medical journey began when Ted went to a doctor to find out why he was having chest pains. I was not too alarmed because, with his knowledge of medicine, Ted was often given to self-diagnosis, and with his brooding Hungarian heritage, he usually arrived at the most horrifying conclusions.

This time, it was angina. Although I tried to suggest that his pain might be coming from something more benign, such as muscular strain, he clung to his grim deduction. He did not want me to go to the doctor with him, and because I was not really worried, I didn't insist.

Thus it was that I called his office from various phone booths until I finally found him in as I went about my business in New York City. As soon as I heard his voice, I knew this time he was right. It *was* angina. Standing on Madison Avenue in an open phone booth, I suddenly felt as if I were on a plane that had hit an air pocket, hurtling me from my seat, my terror escalating with each violent toss.

I don't remember coming home or what we said to each other when we got there. It was clear that he was frightened and angry, and I couldn't find a way to break through the wall those feelings had placed between us. His resistance made me angry as well, not just because my husband might be dangerously ill, but because—and, totally irrationally—I wanted comforting from him. I wanted him to assure me he was going to be all right, that our lives would not change.

Although I have always had my own career as a writer, I then realized how dependent I was on Ted to be there for me, to make me feel protected. I also thought how ironic it was that, in an age when women are so proud of their medical awareness, I was so ignorant of what was happening to Ted. We know all about the diseases we may encounter as we grow older, yet how many of us are really knowledgeable about what may happen to the men in our lives? Long before it happens, we should learn about such conditions as heart disease, prostate cancer, and bypass surgery. If we're lucky, we'll never have to put this knowledge to use, but if suddenly life turns upside down, as mine did with that telephone call, we won't feel so helpless and out of control.

Having caring people around you also helps immeasurably. This is not a time to bravely sit in a hospital waiting room alone. Ted's sister and physician-husband had taken a trip to Russia, not knowing that surgery would be so imminent. When our niece, their married daughter, asked me whether she should try to find them to tell them what was happening, I said I thought that they would want to know. What I didn't consciously realize until they arrived at the hospital two days later (coming straight to the hospital with all their luggage) was how much I wanted them to be there for me. My brother-in-law's medical training made it easier to get some medical information, but more importantly, they loved Ted as I did, and it helped to know that they understood what I was feeling.

Similarly, I did not deny my feelings in front of my young adult children. My normal modus operandi was to protect them from emotional pain, but I could not play a strong role when I was in so much pain myself. From the moment we left Ted in the hospital the night before surgery until he left the building two weeks later, they were, more often than not, at my side as equals in unmitigated pain.

There are different ways that people react to the experience of undergoing bypass surgery. Some are truly exhilarated when they wake up from surgery, feeling grateful that they have been given a new chance at life. This is especially true for people who have suffered from the restrictions of heart disease before surgery.

For Ted, who had been so active, anger and depression were the primary emotions. He felt conspired against by his doctors and family. Left to his own desires, he would not have been operated on, he said. He would have gone about his life as usual and let the chips fall where they may. I was told by dear Dr. Dack that this is not an uncommon reaction, particularly for men. Like a child who wants protection from his mother, a man can blame his wife for his defenseless anguish.

So I became the target of Ted's resentment. I was the one who had allied myself with the doctors instead of with him. I was walking around while he was lying prone on a hospital bed. I was going to have no limitations on my life, whereas he would be a weakened version of the man he used to be.

Friends who witnessed his behavior were amazed, as Ted has always been my proudest supporter. In decades of marriage, there has been hardly any time that we were truly at odds. A friend of mine, who is a psychiatrist, took me out for a drink one day after meeting me at the hospital and expanded on what I had heard from Dr. Dack. In illness, old fears and conflicts over dependence surface, she explained, and are often acted out until the frightening sense of helplessness begins to recede.

If your spouse shows similar behavior, do your best to withstand the emotional blows. They will indeed pass as soon as strength returns and your partner can believe that he or she will not be permanently defenseless.

Dr. Dack has been mentioned several times in this book. I mention him because he was as important to me as he was to Ted. During the six-hour operation, he came down periodically to give me progress bulletins, reassuring me each time that everything was going well. That he was always available for questions was enormously helpful to our family. I urge women, especially, to try to establish a relationship with the cardiologist and surgeon so that you won't feel inhibited about seeking their help. When a doctor holds a person's life in his or her hands, the people in that person's life should be the doctor's patients as well.

Having such a relationship will also help you when you feel some need is being overlooked. On two occasions I felt that Ted was not being given the correct care. One incident involved giving him a drug that had been recommended by a young physician's assistant to stop Ted's breathing difficulties. The nurses and attending physician refused to consider it as it was not on their charts. It was quite late when I called Dr. Dack at home. He had given me the number. Even if you have to call a doctor's answering service, if you say you are calling in an emergency from a hospital, the doctor will undoubtedly call you back. Dr. Dack listened to my report on the suggested drug and agreed to try it instead of the tracheostomy already being planned. The results were successful, and Ted was spared a terrible new trauma. The most important moral of this story is to allow yourself to intervene when you feel there is a need. Even if you are generally nonassertive, this is the time to change behavioral gears.

Out of the hospital, the next few weeks may be a source of shared gratitude and delight, or a time of even darker moods from the recovering patient. Ted was convinced that his life would never be the same. The doctors had told him he would feel so much better. The truth was, he felt so much worse.

During these weeks of recovery, the patient is not allowed to drive a car, or make love, or go to work. Even as the patient protests all these rules, he or she knows that these activities are still too strenuous. It takes great effort not to be contaminated by these dark moods. Your spouse's fears feed into your own. If she winces in some pain or if he takes a suddenly rasping breath, you may be terrified. However, you can be more rational than your partner is during this time, and you have to hang on to that rationality. Read about the condition, talk to the doctors, and try to see the small improvements that she or he is too frightened to observe.

As Ted wrote, three months after his surgery, we were in Italy. A favorite photo from the trip shows us both sitting in the Piazza San Marco. We look healthy and happy.

Especially happy to be together.

Notes

I started writing this book two years after my July 1989 four-vessel bypass surgery. I completed the final chapters in mid-1994. The references were accumulated over a period of three years. These notes were written in late 1995; thus, the reader will note that some of the information is dated, while some is relatively new.

Because diagnostic and interventional cardiology are not static but growing areas of medical science, by the time this book is published and gets into readers' hands, much of what I have said may be out of date. Therefore, I ask the interested reader to take these notes and references as a starting point for his or her own look at what bypass surgery can mean as an option to treat angina or some other coronary artery disease. The fact that some experts believe that 40 percent or more of bypasses should not be done should give every candidate pause before agreeing to surgery.

Books that were helpful to me included:

Michael A. Crouch, M.D., ed., *The Family in Medical Practice* (Springer-Verlag, 1987).
Jeffrey Gold, M.D., and Tony Eprile, *The Well-Informed Patient's Guide to Coronary Bypass Surgery* (Dell, 1990).
Jonathan Halperin, M.D., and Richard Levine, *Bypass* (Times Books, 1985).
Gloria Hochman, *Heart Bypass—What Every Patient Must Know* (St. Martin's Press, 1982).
Larry King, with B.D. Colen, *Mr. King, You're Having A Heart Attack* (Delacorte Press, 1989).
Sigfried Kra, M.D., *Coronary Bypass Surgery—Who Needs It?* (W.W. Norton, 1986).

James A. Pantano, M.D., *Living with Angina* (Harper Perennial, 1990).

Robert Pritikin, *The New Pritikin Program* (Simon & Schuster, 1990).

Jane Schoenberg and JoAnn Stichman, *Heart Family Handbook* (Hanley & Belfus, 1990).

Notes on the Chapters

Chapter 1

Simon Dack, M.D., F.A.C.C., my cardiologist, died in February 1994. There is no question in my mind that his care, skill, and most important to my family, compassion, were responsible for my recovery from surgery. Dr. Dack was the consummate physician. More than that, he was an inspired editor (he was the founding editor of the *American Journal of Cardiology*), investigator, and teacher. In 1994, one of his peers, Charles Fisch, M.D., F.A.C.C., wrote this in his presentation of the American College of Cardiology's Distinguished Service Award to Dr. Dack: "Dr. Dack has been a continuing benefactor to our generation and those that will follow by providing an image for all to see what the profession is all about: scholarly achievement, continuous learning, dedication, legitimacy, and respect for all those who can benefit from the profession's caring."

Chapter 2

"Toward Fewer Procedures and Better Outcomes," *Journal of the American Medical Association* 269, no. 6 (1993): 794–95.

David Lash, M.D., "Coronary Artery Disease: The Latest on Prevention," *Postgraduate Medicine* 91, no. 3 (1992): 179–85.

Carla M. Kingsley and Satyendra C. Gupta, "How to Avoid the Risk of Coronary Artery Disease," *Postgraduate Medicine* 91, no. 4 (1992): 147–60.

Valentin Faustere, M.D., et al., "The Pathogenesis of Coronary Artery Disease and the Acute Coronary Symptoms," *New England Journal of Medicine* 326, no. 5 (1992): 310–17.

"Defusing the Triggers of Heart Attack," *Focus* (February 28, 1991; a newsletter published by Harvard Medical School).

"Coronary Bypass Surgery: How to Avoid It," *HealthFacts* (October 1991; a newsletter published by the Center for Medical Consumers, New York City).

Chapter 3

"America's Best Hospitals," *U.S. News & World Report* (April 30, 1990).

Gail Bronson, "A Consumer's Guide to Making Your Surgery as Painless as Possible," *American Health* (April 1991).

Janice Hopkins Tanne, "How to Be a Savvy Medical Consumer—Finding Good Doctors, Checking Their Credentials, Asking Tough Questions," *New York Magazine* (November 25, 1991).

New York State Department of Health, "Coronary Artery Bypass Surgery in New York State" (December 1993).

Chapter 4

American College of Cardiology/American Heart Association Task Force on Assessment of Diagnostic and Therapeutic Cardiovascular Procedures, "ACC/AHA Guidelines and Indications for Coronary Artery Bypass Surgery," *Journal of the American College of Cardiology* 17, no. 3 (March 1, 1991): 543–89.

H. J. C. Swan, "Guidelines for Judicious Use of Electrocardiography," *Journal of Critical Care Illness* 7, no. 6 (June 1992).

"Exercise Stress Testing for the Family Physician," *American Family Physician* 45 (1992): 121–32.

Jack McCallion and Laurence Krenis, M.D., "Preoperative Cardiac Evaluation," *American Family Physician* 45, no. 4 (April 1992): 1723–32.

American College of Cardiology/American Heart Association Task Force on Assessment of Cardiovascular Procedures (Subcommittee on Exercise Testing), "Guidelines for Exercise Testing," *Journal of the American College of Cardiology* 8, no. 3 (September 1986): 725–38.

American College of Cardiology/American Heart Association Task Force on Assessment of Diagnostic and Therapeutic Cardiovascular Procedures (Subcommittee on Coronary Angiography), "Guidelines for Coronary Angiography," *Journal of the American College of Cardiology* 10, no. 4 (October 1987): 935–50.

"CT Wins Favor in CAD Diagnosis," *Medical World News* (January 1991): 23.

Lawrence M. Fisher, "A Way to Look into the Heart and Detect the Killer Plaque," *New York Times*, August 23, 1992, sec. 3, p. 8.

"A Patient's Guide to Outpatient Cardiac Catheterization," C. R. Bard, 129 Concord Road, Box 566, Billerica, MA 01822, 1989.

Julian Purcell, M.D., "Cardiac Catheterization and Other Cardiac Diagnostic Tests and Radiological Procedures," Pritchett & Hall Associates, 1985.

Chapter 5

Thomas B. Graboys, M.D., *et al.*, "Results of a Second-Opinion Trial among Patients Recommended for Coronary Angiography," *Journal of the American Medical Association* 268, no. 16 (November 11, 1992): 2537–40.

P. J. Walter, M.D., *et al.*, "Quality of Life after Open Heart Surgery," *Quality of Life Research* 1 (1992): 77–83.

"Second Opinions for Surgery—Avoiding Unnecessary Operations, Deaths & Expenses," *Health Letter* (February 1990).

Chapter 7

Cited in this chapter were data from a report based on a survey conducted by the Health Care Finance Administration of 286 hospitals (*Physician's Weekly,* March 4, 1991). The range for bypass without cost of catheterization were $21,092, at Ohio State University Hospital, to $33,671, at Boston's University Hospital. It was estimated that, in 1992, Medicare paid $3.5 billion for 145,000 bypasses. In March 1992, Methodist Hospital in Houston reported to me that the average cost of a single coronary bypass in 1990 was $30,000. That same year, Johns Hopkins told me that the bypass operation (regardless of the number of blockages that are cleared) was $20,000 to $25,000.

Chapter 8

Lee H. Hillborne, *et al.*, "Percutaneous Transluminal Coronary Angioplasty: A Literature Review and Ratings of Appropriateness and Necessity," prepared for the Cardiac Advisory Committee of the State of New York. (Santa Monica, CA: Rand, 1991). This is a literature review of 332 articles (75 percent research), 13 of which reported on randomized clinical trials. The efficacy was judged by relief of angina, prevention of a heart attack, and long-term survival. Restenosis occurred in 25 to 35 percent of patients, most often within six months of the PTCA. About one in five, or 20 percent, of the patients in the studies required repeat PTCA. About 8 to 13 percent had subsequent bypass surgery.

Ted Feldman, M.D., and Mauro Moscucci, M.D., "Update on PTCA: What Are the Limitations? Can They Be Overcome by New Devices?" *Journal of Critical Illness* 8, no. 4 (April 1993): 461–78 (a look at atherectomy, intra-arterial stents, and laser catheters).

American College of Cardiology/American Heart Association, "Guidelines for Percutaneous Transluminal Coronary Angioplasty," *Journal of the American College of Cardiology* 12, no. 2 (August 1988): 529–45.

"Coronary Angioplasty," *Mayo Clinic Health Letter* 11, no. 7 (July 1993).

Patricia L. Cole, M.D., and Ronald J. Krone, M.D., "PTCA Update: Is Your Patient Now a Candidate?" *Journal of Critical Care Illness* 6, no. 1 (February 1991): 166–88.

Chapter 9

Debra V. Owings, et al., "Autologous Blood Donations prior to Elective Cardiac Surgery: Safety and Effect on Subsequent Blood Use," *Journal of the American Medical Association* 262, no. 14 (October 1989): 1963–68.

Chapter 10

Claude M. Grondin, M.D., et al., "Coronary Artery Bypass Grafting with Saphenous Vein," *Circulation* (1989 supp.): 1.24–29.

Floyd D. Loop, M.D., et al., "Influence of the Internal-Mammary Artery Graft on 10-Year Survival and Other Cardiac Events," *New England Journal of Medicine* 314 (1986): 1–6.

Carole A. Gassert, R.N., and Susan G. Burrows, R.N., "Going for Heart Surgery: What You Need to Know" (Atlanta: Pritchett & Hull, 1990).

Gloria Hochman, *Heart Bypass: What Every Patient Must Know* (St. Martin's Press, 1982). This excellent book, though somewhat dated, has valuable information. The section "What Is the Operation Like, and What Are the Risks?" was very helpful.

Chapter 11

Arden Christen, D.D.S., "Bouncing Back from Heart Surgery: Personal Reflections," *Indiana University School of Dentistry Alumni Bulletin* 2 (Fall 1987): 8–13. Dr. Christen, a dentist whom I met in 1981, became a close friend and colleague in my work as an antismoking activist. To get a reprint (well worth the effort), write Dr. Christen at the Indiana University School of Dentistry, in Indianapolis, Indiana 46202.

Chapter 12

"Patients' Rights," New York State Hospital Code Section 405.7.

Chapter 13

There is more written about diet and heart disease than I could share. There is no question that eliminating fat from your diet reduces the risk of suffering from one or more of the symptoms of coronary artery disease. The best books on diet are by Pritikin and Ornish. Also listed are some of the articles I found to be helpful in writing this chapter.

Robert Pritikin, *The New Pritikin Program* (New York: Simon & Schuster, 1990).
Dean M. Ornish, M.D., *Program for Reversing Heart Disease* (Ballantine, 1990).
Etta Saltos, "The Food Pyramid–Food Label Connection," *FDA Consumer* (June 1993): 17–20.
"Medical Essay," a supplement of *Mayo Clinic Health Letter* (June 1993).
Lawrence R. Shapiro, M.D., "More on Chewing the Fat: The Good Fat and the Good Cholesterol," editorial in *New England Journal of Medicine* (December 12, 1994): 1740–41.
Angelo M. Scanu, "Lipoprotein(a): A Genetic Risk Factor for Premature Coronary Heart Disease," *Journal of the American Medical Association* 267, no. 24 (June 24, 1992): 3326–29.

Steven A. Grover, M.D., et al., "The Benefits of Treating Hyperlipidemia to Prevent Coronary Heart Disease: Estimating Changes in Life Expectancy and Morbidity," *Journal of the American Medical Association* 267, no. 6 (February 12, 1992): 816–22.

Chapter 14

James M. Rippe, M.D., et al., "Walking for Health and Fitness," *Journal of the American Medical Association* 259, no. 18 (May 13, 1988): 2720–24.

Fred A. Stutman, M.D., *The Doctor's Walking Book* (New York: Ballantine Books, 1980).

Risteard Mulcahy, M.D., "Beat Heart Disease! A Cardiologist Explains How You Can Help Your Heart and Enjoy a Healthier Life" (New York: Arco, 1979).

Carl J. Lavie, M.D., et al., "Exercise and the Heart—Good, Benign, Or Evil?" *Postgraduate Medicine/Cardiovascular Disease* 91, no. 2 (February 1992).

Timo A. Lakka, M.D., et al., "Relation of Leisure Time Physical Activity and Cardiorespiratory Fitness to the Risk of Acute Myocardial Infarction in Medicine," *New England Journal of Medicine* 330, no. 22 (June 2, 1994): 1549–54.

Glossary

Angina: See Angina pectoris.

Angina pectoris: Not a disease but a symptom of coronary artery disease that is most often characterized by discomfort or pain felt in the chest or the muscles covering the chest (pectorals). Sometimes the pain is mild; sometimes it's severe. Often patients with angina have no pain at all. Sometimes the pain is not in the chest. It may be in the jaw during exercise. The pain is usually caused by constriction of the coronary arteries. It can be started by exercise, physical exertion, or stress, or it can even be of emotional origin. Walking up a steep hill, climbing stairs, and sexual intercourse have all been known to cause angina. You might regard the pain as a call for oxygen by the heart that is not being met due to the narrowing (blockage) of the vessels that supply oxygen-carrying blood to the heart. A spasm of these vessels can also narrow the arteries and cause angina. See also Unstable angina.

Angiograms: The motion pictures produced by angiography.

Angiography: A diagnostic test usually performed to determine if there is any blockage of the arteries that supply blood to the heart (or sometimes the legs). To do the test, an angiographer inserts a small tube (catheter) under fluoroscopic control into the artery, then injects a dye which shows blockages in the vessels.

Angioplasty: The process of inserting a tube, called a catheter, equipped with a special balloon, into a blocked artery to open the artery. Over 500,000 are done in the United States each year.

Atherectomy: A relatively new and still experimental way of using a special device (not unlike a Roto-Rooter) to remove plaque from an artery.

Atheroma: Material (consisting in part of cholesterol and other lipoproteins) which forms on the walls of arteries, reducing blood flow. Also called plaque.

Atherosclerosis: A disease of the lining of the vessels that transport blood, in the course of which the deposit of atheromatous material (including cholesterol) causes the vessel to narrow (hardening of the arteries), reducing the flow of blood.

Balloon angioplasty: See Angioplasty.

Beta blocker: A class of prescription medicines used to treat hypertension and the pain of angina.

Blood lipid analysis: The process of determining the amount of various fatty substances (lipids) in the blood.

Blood pressure: The force of the blood against the walls of arteries, the vessels that carry blood away from the heart.

Board-certified: A term used to describe a physician who has passed examinations established by a medical specialty board. Not all physicians are board-certified, but everyone who has been board-certified is a physician. Specialty organizations frequently require a physician to show evidence of taking continuing medical education courses in order to retain his or her certification.

Bypass surgery: An operation performed to treat angina, in which vessels are taken from a person and used to bypass her or his blocked coronary arteries. Also called a coronary artery bypass graft (CABG).

CABG: Coronary artery bypass graft. See Bypass surgery.

CAD: See Coronary artery disease.

Calcium antagonist: A class of medications used to treat hypertension and angina.

Cardiac catheterization: A surgical procedure that involves inserting a special tube (catheter) into the vessels that supply blood to the heart. Used in coronary arteriography as an X-ray procedure to examine the arteries that supply blood to the heart.

Cardiac intensive care unit (CICU): A specially equipped hospital room or area which provides twenty-four-hour care to patients who have suffered heart attacks or who have undergone heart surgery. Brightly lit, noisy, and often operating at a frenetic pace, the CICU is where a bypass patient is taken following surgery. This is where the patient will remain until the surgeon believes he or she can breathe without mechanical assistance and no longer requires intensive, around-the-clock monitoring of vital functions. Seeing a loved one in the CICU immediately after a bypass is likely to cause concern to the family because the patient will be unconscious, with tubes stuck in both natural and surgically made openings. It is not a pretty sight and is certainly unsuitable for anyone who becomes queasy easily.

Cardiologist: A physician who specializes in the treatment of patients with diseases of the heart.

Cardiopulmonary bypass: A machine or pump that is used in open-heart and bypass surgery to provide the body with blood. The machine bypasses the heart and lungs so that the heart remains still for the surgery.

Cholesterol: A fatty substance that can cause blockage of arteries (and is also a major component of gallstones). Most of the cholesterol in our bodies is produced by the liver, but some is absorbed from fat-containing foods.

CICU: See Cardiac intensive care unit (CICU).

Computed tomography (CT): A method for measuring calcification in arteries.

Coronary artery bypass graft (CABG): See Bypass surgery.

Coronary artery disease (CAD): An illness resulting from a blockage of the vessels that bring blood to the heart. There are three major vessels; the right and the two branches of the left main artery—the left circumflex and the left descending.

Coronary artery stenosis: A narrowing of the vessels that take blood away from the heart.

Coronary risk factors: Usually refers to characteristics typical of people who have coronary artery disease. Among them are some that can be avoided (smoking); some that can be treated by diet, exercise, and medication (high cholesterol level, hypertension, diabetes); and some no one can do anything about (gender or family history of heart disease or both).

Coronary Spasm: A temporary narrowing of an artery that occurs when the patient is at rest. The reasons for coronary spasm are not well understood.

ECG: See Electrocardiogram (ECG).

Echocardiograms: Pictures of the heart produced by echocardiography (use of high-frequency sound). Used in the diagnosis of heart disease.

Ejection fraction: The amount of blood, expressed in percentage terms, that is ejected from the heart's left chamber (ventricle) at each heartbeat. An ejection fraction of less than 50 percent usually indicates some damage to the heart muscle.

EKG: See Electrocardiogram (ECG).

Electrocardiogram (ECG): A recording of the electrical activity of the heart that is used to diagnose heart disease. Also abbreviated EKG.

Exercise tolerance test: Also called a stress test. Usually based on the twenty-one-minute Bruce Exercise Protocol, whereby the patient walks on a treadmill while monitored by an ECG machine. The test starts with a warm-up at 1.7 mph on a 5 percent grade. Both the speed and the grade are subsequently increased according to a formula based on the age, weight, and response of the patient's heart (as measured by changes in blood pressure and rate of heartbeats). The increases run from Stage 1 (walking at 1.7 mph on a 10 percent grade) to Stage 4 (walking a 4.2 mph on a 16 percent grade). Stage 4 is where most patients with coronary artery disease will report discomfort or pain or both. If this does not happen and there are no abnormal changes in heart rate, the test may be continued to Stage 7, where the patient is running on a 22 percent grade. One of the key indicators used in expressing exercise tolerance test results is maximal normal heart rate, which can be calculated by subtracting the patient's age from 220. Thus, a sixty-year-old man in good health would never be expected to exceed 160 beats per minute.

Fatty acid: The building blocks of fats. A molecule composed of mostly carbon and hydrogen atoms.

Fluoroscopy: A technique in which X-rays are used to visualize internal structures.

Glucose: A form of sugar that occurs in fruits and honey.

HDL: See High-density lipoproteins (HDL).

Heart attack: Popular term used to describe what happens when a portion of the heart muscle dies because its supply of oxygen-carrying blood is totally blocked. The medical term for it is myocardial infarction. About 700,000 people with heart attacks are hospitalized each year in the United States. About 75,000 deaths are attributed to heart attacks. According to some cardiologists, 15,000 of these deaths could have been prevented if "clot-buster" drugs were widely used after the attack. Drugs such as streptokinase and tissue plasminogen activator (TPA) are most often used.

High-density lipoproteins (HDL): Fatty substances that can remove cholesterol from the blood. Current medical thinking is that the "good" cholesterol, HDL, can reduce the risk of heart attacks by reducing the amount of cholesterol deposited on the walls of arteries.

Hypercholesterolemia: Excessive amount of cholesterol in blood.

Isotopes: Forms of a chemical element with slightly different atomic mass and chemical properties. Although the term has become associated with radioactivity, that is not exactly true because many familiar chemical elements have nonradioactive isotopes.

Lasers: Devices that use generated ultrahigh-frequency light. Surgical lasers are used to raise the temperature at the tip of a tiny probe to where it can burn, or "bake," tissue.

LDL: See Low-density lipoproteins (LDL).

Lipids: Any one of a group of fats, including cholesterol and triglycerides.

Low-density lipoproteins (LDL): Fatty substances that carry cholesterol through the bloodstream. The "bad" cholesterol.

Met: Metabolic equivalent. A measure of physical activity.

MUGA: See Multiple gated acquisition (MUGA) test.

Multiple gated acquisition (MUGA) test: Also called a nuclear scan. A test used to measure the efficiency of the heart by measuring its contractibility. A radioisotope (usually thallium-201) is injected into a conscious patient so that a special camera can record heart contractions. The information goes to a computer that calculates the percentage of efficiency, expressed as the ejection fraction. When the ejection fraction is below 75 percent, physicians will seek ways to raise it. See also Ejection fraction.

Myocardial infarction: See Heart attack.

Nitroglycerin: A chemical patented by Alfred Nobel in 1864 that is used to make dynamite and which, under the name of amyl nitrite, has also been used for over one hundred years to treat angina. It is available in the form of tablets, transdermal patches, and sublingual lozenges containing various doses.

NMR: Nuclear magnetic resonance. See Multiple gated acquisition (MUGA) test.

Nuclear imaging agent: A radioactive substance which, when injected in tiny amounts, can be used to visualize tissues and internal structures.

Nuclear magnetic resonance (NMR) scan: See Multiple gated acquisition (MUGA) test.

Nuclear scan: See Multiple gated acquisition (MUGA) test.

Occlusion: The total blockage of an artery.

Open-heart surgery: Any operation when the cardiopulmonary bypass (heart-lung) machine is used.

Percutaneous transluminal coronary angioplasty (PTCA): A procedure in which a catheter containing a balloon is inserted into a blocked artery and inflated one or more times to open the artery.

PTCA: See Percutaneous transluminal coronary angioplasty (PTCA).

Quality of life: A measurement of the outcome of treatment. There are at least two dimensions. Functional status and well-being. Function refers to things a patient can or can't do. Vitality and lack of pain are both associated with a person's well-being.

Radioisotopes: Radioactive substances (variant forms of chemical elements) used to help visualize tissues and internal structures. Radioactive thallium is a frequently used radioisotope because of its special affinity for heart muscle, which will start absorbing it within minutes after an injection. A scan of the heart will then show if the muscle is absorbing less than usual of the radioisotope. This would indicate damage and some loss of heart function.

Restenosis: The closing of a bypass graft or artery that was opened by surgical means. Stenosis is derived from a Greek term for narrowing.

Saphenous vein: A blood vessel in the upper leg which can be removed to provide material for a bypass. One end is attached to the aorta; the other end is attached below a blocked part of an artery that carries blood away from the heart.

S-T segment: A measurement of heart activity, shown on the record of an ECG. Any abnormality usually indicates the presence of coronary artery disease.

Saturated fat: Any fat that can increase the cholesterol level. Present in animal-origin foods such as butter and milk, and in vegetable-origin foods such as palm oils and hydrogenated shortenings.

Stents: Devices inserted into a blood vessel to keep it open.

Stress tests: See Exercise tolerance test.

Transluminal angioplasty: A diagnostic procedure whereby a catheter is passed through a vessel (lumen).

Unstable angina: Chest discomfort or pain that occurs when a person is at rest. Unstable angina is different and more serious than stable angina. It is characterized by anginal discomfort when resting, and the pain often awakens patients from sleep. It occurs suddenly on exertion. It has been estimated that more than 1 million Americans have unstable angina. It causes more than 830,000 hospitalizations a year. Health care costs are estimated at several billion dollars a year.

Urethra: The tube which carries urine away from the bladder.

Visiting privileges: The granting of permission to a physician who is not on a hospital's staff to visit, or even to operate, on a patient. When a physician does not have visiting privileges, he or she will not be permitted such access.

Index